# PET Imaging of Brain Tumors

*Editors*

SANDIP BASU
WEI CHEN

# PET CLINICS

www.pet.theclinics.com

*Consulting Editor*
ABASS ALAVI

April 2013 • Volume 8 • Number 2

ELSEVIER

1600 John F. Kennedy Boulevard • Suite 1800 • Philadelphia, Pennsylvania, 19103-2899

http://www.theclinics.com

**PET CLINICS Volume 8, Number 2**
**April 2013 ISSN 1556-8598, ISBN-13: 978-1-4557-7139-4**

Editor: Adrianne Brigido

**Photocopying**

Single photocopies of single articles may be made for personal use as allowed by national copyright laws. Permission of the Publisher and payment of a fee is required for all other photocopying, including multiple or systematic copying, copying for advertising or promotional purposes, resale, and all forms of document delivery. Special rates are available for educational institutions that wish to make photocopies for non-profit educational classroom use. For information on how to seek permission visit www.elsevier.com/permissions or call: (+44) 1865 843830 (UK)/(+1) 215 239 3804 (USA).

**Derivative Works**

Subscribers may reproduce tables of contents or prepare lists of articles including abstracts for internal circulation within their institutions. Permission of the Publisher is required for resale or distribution outside the institution. Permission of the Publisher is required for all other derivative works, including compilations and translations (please consult www.elsevier.com/permissions).

**Electronic Storage or Usage**

Permission of the Publisher is required to store or use electronically any material contained in this journal, including any article or part of an article (please consult www.elsevier.com/permissions). Except as outlined above, no part of this publication may be reproduced, stored in a retrieval system or transmitted in any form or by any means, electronic, mechanical, photocopying, recording or otherwise, without prior written permission of the Publisher.

**Notice**

No responsibility is assumed by the Publisher for any injury and/or damage to persons or property as a matter of products liability, negligence or otherwise, or from any use or operation of any methods, products, instructions or ideas contained in the material herein. Because of rapid advances in the medical sciences, in particular, independent verification of diagnoses and drug dosages should be made. Although all advertising material is expected to conform to ethical (medical) standards, inclusion in this publication does not constitute a guarantee or endorsement of the quality or value of such product or of the claims made of it by its manufacturer.

*PET Clinics* (ISSN 1556-8598) is published quarterly by Elsevier Inc., 360 Park Avenue South, New York, NY 10010-1710. Months of issue are January, April, July, and October. Periodicals postage paid at New York, NY, and additional mailing offices. Subscription prices per year are $215.00 (US individuals), $309.00 (US institutions), $110.00 (US students), $244.00 (Canadian individuals), $345.00 (Canadian institutions), $134.00 (Canadian students), $260.00 (foreign individuals), $345.00 (foreign institutions), and $134.00 (foreign students). To receive student and resident rate, orders must be accompanied by name of affiliated institution, date of term, and the signature of program/residency coordinator on institution letterhead. Orders will be billed at individual rate until proof of status is received. Foreign air speed delivery is included in all Clinics subscription prices. All prices are subject to change without notice. POSTMASTER: Send address changes to PET Clinics, Elsevier Health Sciences Division, Subscription Customer Service, 3251 Riverport Lane, Maryland Heights, MO 63043. **Customer Service: 1-800-654-2452 (U.S. and Canada); 314-447-8871 (outside U.S. and Canada). Fax: 314-447-8029. E-mail: journalscustomerservice-usa@elsevier.com (for print support); journalsonlinesupport-usa@elsevier.com (for online support).**

*Reprints.* For copies of 100 or more of articles in this publication, please contact the Commercial Reprints Department, Elsevier Inc., 360 Park Avenue South, New York, NY 10010-1710. Tel.: 212-633-3812; Fax: 212-462-1935; E-mail: reprints@elsevier.com.

Printed and bound by CPI Group (UK) Ltd, Croydon, CR0 4YY

Transferred to digital print 2013

# Contributors

## CONSULTING EDITOR

**ABASS ALAVI, MD, PhD (Hon), DSc (Hon)**
Professor of Radiology, Division of Nuclear
Medicine, University of Pennsylvania School of
Medicine; Department of Radiology, Hospital
of the University of Pennsylvania, Philadelphia,
Pennsylvania

## EDITORS

**SANDIP BASU, MBBS (Hons), DRM, DNB**
MNAMS, Radiation Medicine Centre, Bhabha
Atomic Research Centre, Tata Memorial
Hospital Annexe, Parel, Bombay, India

**WEI CHEN, MD**
Department of Molecular and Medical
Pharmacology, David Geffen School of
Medicine, University of California Los Angeles,
Los Angeles, California

## AUTHORS

**WEI CHEN, MD**
Department of Molecular and Medical
Pharmacology, David Geffen School of
Medicine, University of California Los Angeles,
Los Angeles, California

**TIMOTHY F. CLOUGHESY, MD**
Department of Neurology, David Geffen School
of Medicine, University of California Los
Angeles, Los Angeles, California

**JOHANNES CZERNIN, MD**
Department of Molecular and Medical
Pharmacology, David Geffen School of
Medicine, University of California Los Angeles,
Los Angeles, California

**MAARTEN L. DONSWIJK, MD**
Department of Radiology and Nuclear
Medicine, University Medical Center Utrecht,
Utrecht, The Netherlands

**VINCENT DUNET, BSc, MD**
Departments of Nuclear Medicine and
Radiology, Lausanne University, Lausanne,
Switzerland

**BENJAMIN M. ELLINGSON, PhD**
Assistant Professor, Departments of
Radiological Sciences, Biomedical Physics
and Biomedical Engineering, David Geffen
School of Medicine, University of California
Los Angeles, Los Angeles, California

**ROBERT J. HARRIS, BS**
Departments of Radiological Sciences and
Biomedical Physics, David Geffen School of
Medicine, University of California Los Angeles,
Los Angeles, California

**KRISZTIAN HOMICSKO, MD, PhD**
Department of Medical Oncology, Lausanne
University Hospital, Lausanne, Switzerland

**ANDREAS F. HOTTINGER, MD, PhD**
Department of Clinical Neurosciences,
Lausanne University Hospital, Lausanne,
Switzerland

**SARAH N. KHAN, MD**
Department of Radiological Sciences, David
Geffen School of Medicine, University of
California Los Angeles, Los Angeles, California

**THOMAS C. KWEE, MD, PhD**
Department of Radiology and Nuclear Medicine, University Medical Center Utrecht, Utrecht, The Netherlands

**ALBERT LAI, MD, PhD**
Department of Neurology, David Geffen School of Medicine, University of California Los Angeles, Los Angeles, California

**MARC LEVIVIER, MD, PhD**
Professor, Department of Clinical Neurosciences, Lausanne University Hospital, Lausanne, Switzerland

**MICHAEL LINETSKY, MD**
Assistant Professor, Department of Radiological Sciences, David Geffen School of Medicine, University of California Los Angeles, Los Angeles, California

**JONATHAN McCONATHY, MD, PhD**
Assistant Professor of Radiology, Divisions of Nuclear Medicine and Radiological Sciences, Mallinckrodt Institute of Radiology, St Louis, Missouri

**LAURA NEGRETTI, MD**
Department of Radiation Therapy, Lausanne University Hospital, Lausanne, Switzerland

**PHIOANH L. NGHIEMPHU, MD**
Department of Neurology, David Geffen School of Medicine, University of California Los Angeles, Los Angeles, California

**MICHAEL E. PHELPS, PhD**
Department of Molecular and Medical Pharmacology, David Geffen School of Medicine, University of California Los Angeles, Los Angeles, California

**WHITNEY B. POPE, MD, PhD**
Associate Professor of Radiology, Department of Radiological Sciences, David Geffen School of Medicine, University of California Los Angeles, Los Angeles, California

**JOHN O. PRIOR, PhD, MD**
Professor and Head of Department, Department of Nuclear Medicine, Lausanne University Hospital, Lausanne, Switzerland

**SRINIVASAN SENTHAMIZHCHELVAN, PhD**
The Russell H. Morgan Department of Radiology and Radiological Science, Johns Hopkins University School of Medicine, Baltimore, Maryland

**AKASH SHARMA, MD**
Assistant Professor of Radiology, Division of Nuclear Medicine, Mallinckrodt Institute of Radiology, St Louis, Missouri

**ROGER STUPP, MD**
Professor, Department of Clinical Neurosciences, Lausanne University Hospital, Lausanne, Switzerland

**HABIB ZAIDI, PhD, PD**
Division of Nuclear Medicine and Molecular Imaging, Geneva University Hospital; Geneva Neuroscience Center, Geneva University, Geneva, Switzerland; Department of Nuclear Medicine and Molecular Imaging, University Medical Center Groningen, University of Groningen, Groningen, The Netherlands

# Contents

# PET CLINICS

## PROGRAM OBJECTIVE:
The goal of the PET Clinics is to keep practicing radiologists and radiology residents up to date with current clinical practice inpositron emission tomography by providing timely articles reviewing the state of the art in patient care.

## TARGET AUDIENCE:
Practicing radiologists, radiology residents, and other health care professionals who provide patient care utilizing radiologic findings.

## LEARNING OBJECTIVES
Upon completion of this activity, participants will be able to:
1. Review PET parametic response mapping for clinical monitoring and treatment response evaluation in brain tumors.
2. Recognize advanced MRI techniques and their evolving role of PET-MRI in neuro-oncology.
3. Utilize MRI imaging of Glioma in the era of anti-angiogenic therapy.

## ACCREDITATION
The Elsevier Office of Continuing Medical Education (EOCME) is accredited by the Accreditation Council for Continuing Medical Education (ACCME) to provide continuing medical education for physicians.

The EOCME designates this journal-based CME activity for a maximum of 7 *AMA PRA Category 1 Credit*(s)™. Physicians should claim only the credit commensurate with the extent of their participation in the activity.

All other health care professionals completing continuing education credit for this activity will be issued a certificate of participation.

## DISCLOSURE OF CONFLICTS OF INTEREST
The EOCME assesses conflict of interest with its instructors, faculty, planners, and other individuals who are in a position to control the content of CME activities. All relevant conflicts of interest that are identified are thoroughly vetted by EOCME for fair balance, scientific objectivity, and patient care recommendations. EOCME is committed to providing its learners with CME activities that promote improvements or quality in healthcare and not a specific proprietary business or a commercial interest.

**The planning committee, staff, authors and editors listed below have identified no financial relationships or relationships to products or devices they or their spouse/life partner have with commercial interest related to the content of this CME activity:**
Abass Alavi, MD; Sandip Basu, MD; Adrianne Brigido; Wei Chen, MD; Timothy F. Cloughesy, MD; Nicole Congleton; Maarten Donswijk, MSc; Vincent Dunet, MD; Benjamin M. Ellingson, PhD, Ms; Robert J. Harris, BS; Krisztian Homicsko, MD, PhD; Andreas Hottinger, MD, PhD; Sarah N. Khan, MD; Thomas C. Kwee, MD; Sandy Lavery; Marc Levivier, MD, PhD; Michael Linetsky, MD; Jill McNair; Jonathan McConathy, MD, PhD; Mahalakshmi Narayanan; Laura Negretti, MD; Phioanh Nghiemphu, MD; John O. Prior, MD, PhD; Srinivasan Senthamizhchelvan, PhD; Akash Sharma, MD; Roger Stupp, MD; and Habib Zaidi, PhD.

**The planning committee, staff, authors and editors listed below have identified financial relationships or relationships to products or devices they or their spouse/life partner have with commercial interest related to the content of this CME activity:**
Johannes Czernin, MD has stock ownership in Sofie Biosciences.
Albert Lai, MD, PhD has a research grant from Genentech.
Michael E. Phelps, PhD and spouse/partner are on speakers bureau and have stock ownership in Sofie Biosciences.
Whitney Pope, MD, PhD has research grants from Genentech/Roche, Amgen and Tocagen.

## UNAPPROVED/OFF-LABEL USE DISCLOSURE
The EOCME requires CME faculty to disclose to the participants:
1. When products or procedures being discussed are off-label, unlabelled, experimental, and/or investigational (not US Food and Drug Administration (FDA) approved); and
2. Any limitations on the information presented, such as data that are preliminary or that represent ongoing research, interim analyses, and/or unsupported opinions. Faculty may discuss information about pharmaceutical agents that is outside of FDA-approved labelling. This information is intended solely for CME and is not intended to promote off-label use of these medications. If you have any questions, contact the medical affairs department of the manufacturer for the most recent prescribing information.

## TO ENROLL
To enroll in the *PET Clinics* Continuing Medical Education program, call customer service at 1-800-654-2452 or sign up online at http://www.theclinics.com/home/cme. The CME program is available to subscribers for an additional annual fee of $212 USD.

## METHOD OF PARTICIPATION
In order to claim credit, participants must complete the following:
1. Complete enrolment as indicated above.
2. Read the activity.
3. Complete the CME Test and Evaluation. Participants must achieve a score of 70% on the test. All CME Tests and Evaluations must be completed online.

## CME INQUIRIES/SPECIAL NEEDS
For all CME inquiries or special needs, please contact elsevierCME@elsevier.com.

# PET Imaging in Glioma
## The Neuro-Oncologist's Expectations

Andreas F. Hottinger, MD, PhD[a], Marc Levivier, MD, PhD[a],
Laura Negretti, MD[b], Krisztian Homicsko, MD, PhD[c],
Roger Stupp, MD[a],*

## KEYWORDS

- PET • Brain tumor • Glioma • Neuro-oncology • Imaging

## KEY POINTS

- Noninvasive imaging is essential for the precise diagnosis and follow-up of patients with brain tumors.
- PET can play a key role in determining tumor aggressiveness, in determining the optimal biopsy site in low-grade glioma, and in differentiating tumor recurrence from treatment-induced alterations.
- Validation of PET in prospective clinical studies is hampered by lack of reimbursement. For routine clinical use, these techniques would benefit from multicentric studies to establish the exact sensitivity and specificity of the methods, compared with the current standard practices.
- PET imaging needs to be implemented in clinical pathways, and registries should accumulate evidences on whether it results in treatment modifications and improved patient outcome. To this aim, the help of regulating authorities and institutions is needed.

## INTRODUCTION

Management of primary brain tumors and in particular glioma is a complex multidisciplinary exercise. The infiltrative nature of glioma does not allow one to easily demarcate tumor from normal tissue. Tumor location, that is, proximity to eloquent areas, does not permit resection with large safety margins, and radiation therapy is limited by the tolerance of normal brain tissue. Brain is protected by the blood–brain barrier (BBB), and many chemotherapeutic or targeted agents do not reach the tumor cells in adequate concentrations. In high-grade tumors, imaging is facilitated by contrast enhancement, reflecting disruption of the BBB, whereas low-grade glioma usually does not show contrast uptake. However, the absence of enhancement does not exclude a higher-grade tumor.

Virtually all patients will present with tumor progression or recurrence, even after complete resection, followed by radiotherapy and chemotherapy.[1] In low-grade glioma, watchful waiting and repeated clinical and radiological monitoring is commonly the favored approach in younger patients.[2] Adequate and early identification of tumor growth acceleration, malignant transformation, tumor progression, or recurrence is important to determine antitumor therapy.

The evaluation of treatment effect is challenging. Tumor response may be slow and delayed. Residual and recurrent tumor cannot easily be distinguished from treatment response with tumor necrosis and scar tissue, which is also a major impediment to drug development. Early measurable surrogate end points rather than only survival are needed in clinical trials and daily practice.

[a] Department of Clinical Neurosciences, Lausanne University Hospital, Rue du Bugnon 46, Lausanne 1011, Switzerland; [b] Department of Radiation Therapy, Lausanne University Hospital, Rue du Bugnon 46, Lausanne 1011, Switzerland; [c] Department of Medical Oncology, Lausanne University Hospital, Rue du Bugnon 46, Lausanne 1011, Switzerland
* Corresponding author. Department of Clinical Neurosciences, Lausanne University Hospital (CHUV), Rue du Bugnon 46, Lausanne 1011, Switzerland.
E-mail address: roger.stupp@chuv.ch

PET Clin 8 (2013) 117–128
http://dx.doi.org/10.1016/j.cpet.2012.09.006
1556-8598/13/$ – see front matter © 2013 Elsevier Inc. All rights reserved.

In particular low-grade tumors, in which median survival duration is more than 7 to 10 years, require reliable evaluation of treatment effect by imaging.

## MAGNETIC RESONANCE (MR) IMAGING

Magnetic resonance (MR) imaging remains the gold standard for brain tumor imaging. This technique is nowadays universally available and allows excellent and detailed anatomic representation of all brain structures and alterations. The acquisition time usually lasts less than 20 to 30 minutes and can answer most of the clinical questions and situations. Standard T1- and T2-weighted sequences, along with proton-weighted, diffusion-weighted, and perfusion-weighted images, detect and characterize brain tumors. MR imaging also provides additional information about secondary phenomena such as necrosis, intratumoral hemorrhage, edema, or mass effect. MR spectroscopy is used for quantification of several molecules of interest including creatine, choline, and N-acetylaspartate, or less often, lipids or lactates within a selected area of the brain. The relative distribution of these molecules may help to estimate tumor aggressiveness and to differentiate tumor from necrosis or other abnormalities.[3] However, MR spectroscopy has poor spatial resolution and is sensitive to artifacts induced by the proximity of bone, cerebrospinal fluid, or surgical devices.

MR imaging has several limitations: fibrotic changes, scar tissue, contrast enhancement after surgery, or tumor necrosis after radiation therapy cannot be easily differentiated from recurrent or residual tumor.[4,5] MR imaging also has a low sensitivity to differentiate between neoplastic diseases and vascular or inflammatory processes. MR spectroscopy is susceptible to technical variability and artifacts depending on the tumor location. Evaluation and quantification are complicated because often both viable and necrotic tumor tissue are present, especially because of the poor spatial resolution of MR spectroscopy.

## PET SCAN IN NEURO-ONCOLOGY

PET is an imaging technique that allows the noninvasive localization and quantification of physiologic and molecular processes.[6,7] Molecules marked with positron-emitting radionuclides are used in small (diagnostic) doses. These molecules reflect the metabolic process, which can then be measured. PET with specific radioactive tracers provides information on tumor metabolism and growth. Coregistration and image fusion with MR imaging allows adequate correlation with the anatomic structures. PET allows identification of active tumor tissue and a semiquantitative analysis. Repeated PET can be used to follow tumor activity and may allow early documentation of response or recurrence.[8–10] Depending on the organ and clinical questions, various tracers have been developed; selected tracers are briefly discussed in the following sections.

### FDG-PET

Starting in the early 1980s, PET imaging has been investigated for its potential role in the evaluation of brain tumors before and after treatment. $^{18}$F-fluorodeoxy-glucose (FDG) was shown to be actively transported across the BBB into the cells and high FDG uptake usually correlates with a higher tumor grade.[11,12] The first studies with patients investigated the role of FDG-PET in helping to determine the tumor grade. For example, it was shown that FDG-PET was more accurate than contrast computed tomography (CT) for tumor grading.[13] A study evaluating 45 patients with high-grade gliomas after surgery, radiation therapy, and chemotherapy demonstrated that poorly differentiated tumors showed significantly higher FDG uptake than more differentiated ones. An uptake ratio greater than 1.4 compared with the contralateral healthy brain parenchyma was associated with poor prognosis (median survival of 1.9 months vs 19 months if the ratio was <1.4).[14] FDG-PET was shown to be superior to contrast-enhanced CT in identifying early recurrence and predicted outcomes better than the pathologic analysis of biopsies. Moreover, in this study, most patients (19 of 20) with hypermetabolic lesions in areas of previous tumor resection had early tumor recurrence, as confirmed on subsequent follow-up. In all 12 patients with hypometabolic abnormalities, follow-up confirmed the presence of radiation necrosis.[15]

In brain tumors, FDG-PET has several limitations[16,17]: because normal brain tissue shows a high rate of glucose consumption, tumors with only a modest increase in glucose metabolism, such as low-grade tumors, may be difficult to identify. In low-grade gliomas, uptake of FDG may be similar to that in normal white matter, and uptake in high-grade gliomas may be lower than or similar to that of normal gray matter.[18] Moreover, after treatment, FDG uptake may be severely decreased despite persistence of viable tumor tissue.[11]

Coregistration of FDG-PET with MR imaging allows better spatial resolution and anatomic correlation and has been shown to improve the diagnostic performance.[19] MR imaging allows to better delineate the area of interest, whereby any increase of FDG uptake above the expected background level should be considered recurrent tumor. However, because of the overall high glucose consumption in the brain and the consequent lack of sufficient contrast between tumor and normal tissue, FDG-PET is rarely useful in primary brain tumors,[20] with the notable exception of primary central nervous system (CNS) lymphoma.

## Amino Acid PET Tracers

Amino acids are transported into cells by carrier-mediated processes.[21] Amino acid uptake is generally increased in malignant transformation. This increase has been postulated to be linked to increased transport of the amino acids, because of upregulated amino acid transporters, which results in increased flux of the amino acids or/and increased amino acid metabolism (Table 1).[22–24] Amino acid transport is generally accepted to be the rate-limiting step. Increased proliferative activity is linked to increased amino acid transport during all phases of the cell cycle independent of increased vascular permeability.[25,26]

The most significant advantage of these tracers is related to their markedly lower background activity in normal brain tissue compared with FDG, giving a high tumor to normal tissue contrast and enabling the detection of smaller tumors (primary or recurrent). Uptake of amino acids such as tyrosine in brain tumors may be linked to a combination of (1) breakdown of the BBB, (2) upregulation of amino acid transport, and (3) protein synthesis. In contrast, methionine uptake is related to membrane transport phenomena because blockage of protein synthesis does not seem to influence methionine uptake.[27] Nevertheless, [11]C-methionine (MET) was the first amino acid to be evaluated for metabolic brain imaging. Because of the short life of [11]C, necessitating an on-site cyclotron, [18]F-based aromatic amino acid analogs have been developed, which have a significantly longer half-life (110 minutes) allowing distribution to remote centers. For instance, [18]F-labeled aromatic amino acid analogs, including [18]F-fluoro-ethyl-L-tyrosine (FET) has been developed and shown to have similar uptake in brain tumors as MET.[28,29] Tracers others than amino acid analogs have been studied in brain tumors. [18]F-fluoro-L-thymidine (FLT) is a desoxyribonucleotide analog that is not integrated into DNA but taken up into proliferating cells with increased thymidine kinase activity.[30,31]

Compared to other imaging techniques, the spatial resolution of PET imaging remains limited (typically 2–6 mm) in precisely identifying neuroanatomical landmarks. This limitation has been overcome by fusing the images with morphologic imaging modalities that provide a better spatial resolution, such as CT or MR imaging. Moreover, PET is logistically more demanding than MR imaging because there are fewer centers able to perform the examinations. A cyclotron is required to create the radioisotope, which needs to be on-site for the [11]C-based radioisotopes (20 minutes) or within 3 half-lives from a distribution center for [18]F-based radioisotopes (110 minutes). Patient scheduling is more complicated, and the examination time in the scanner may be longer for the patient (40–60 minutes) (Box 1).

## ROLE OF PET IN DETECTING TUMORS AND DIFFERENTIATION FROM OTHER LESIONS

The neuro-oncologist often faces the challenge of determining whether a newly identified brain lesion is malignant or not. In a study of 88 adults with neurologic deficits, FET uptake was shown to have a high sensitivity (93%) for detecting malignant brain lesions, suggesting that a lesion that does not take up FET is unlikely to be tumoral (Fig. 1). However, negative results with FET-PET does not exclude the presence of

**Table 1**
**PET radiopharmaceuticals used in neuro-oncology and targeted molecular processes**

| Tracer | Abbreviation | Biomarker |
| --- | --- | --- |
| [18]F-Fluorodeoxyglucose | FDG | Glucose metabolism |
| [11]C-Methionine | MET | Amino acid transport |
| [18]F-Fluorothyrosine | FET | Amino acid transport |
| [18]F-Fluoro-DOPA | FDOPA | Amino acid transport |
| [18]F-Fluorthymidine | FLT | Proliferation |
| [18]F-Fluormisonidazol | FMISO | Hypoxia |

---

**Box 1**
**Key neuro-oncologic issues that might be addressed by PET**

The role of PET imaging has been mainly investigated in patients with gliomas, as these represent the most frequent and most challenging brain tumors to treat. Management of these tumors includes some specific challenges, where the addition of PET imaging may provide additional information that cannot be reliably obtained by standard MR imaging techniques. These clinical needs include

• **Definition of tumor extent**

For the correct planning of treatment, it is essential that the neurosurgeon and the radiation therapist be able to evaluate as precisely as possible the maximal extent of the tumor and its relationship to neighboring eloquent neurologic structures. This precise evaluation should allow for maximal safe resection of the tumor and for ensuring that the entire tumor or tumor bed is included within the field of radiation therapy.

• **Planning of stereotactic biopsy**

A major challenge of stereotactic biopsy is to ensure that the sample obtained represents adequately the underlying tumor. Histologic classification of the tumor is based on the most aggressive part of the tumor. In tumors suspected of lower-grade gliomas, PET imaging might ensure that the most aggressive metabolically active part of the tumor is being targeted with the biopsy, especially when there is no contrast enhancement on MR imaging.

• **Establishing the prognosis for a specific patient**

Several prognostic factors have been identified including type and grade of tumor, performance status, age, and molecular markers. PET imaging may further help to better predict the outcome and to define a patient's individual prognosis.

• **Assessing response to treatment**

A correct and early assessment of the effect of a therapy on the tumor is essential because it ensures that a therapy is pursued for as long as it is effective and that the treatment may be discontinued as soon as the tumor has become resistant to it.

• **Differentiation of posttreatment effects from tumor progression**

This question is of key importance to differentiate progression or recurrence of disease versus treatment-induced changes in the normal brain parenchyma such as radiation necrosis, pseudoprogression, or postoperative changes.

---

a low-grade glioma or gliomatosis.[32] A recent meta-analysis of 13 studies confirmed the high specificity and sensitivity of abnormal FET uptake in primary brain tumors.[33] This result, based on retrospective analysis of studies with varying inclusion criteria and limited number of patients, however, needs to be validated in prospective studies.

## ROLE OF PET IN DETERMINING THE MOST ADEQUATE SITE FOR STEREOTACTIC BIOPSY IN LOW-GRADE GLIOMAS

Stereotactic biopsies are a frequent tool for establishing the diagnosis of a primary brain tumor. However, the millimeter-small tissue sample may not necessarily be representative of all the characteristics of a large tumor. In high-grade tumors, the biopsy targets contrast enhancement, whereas in low-grade tumors, the location and target center of the biopsy is not easily defined. Standard MR imaging may not identify heterogeneity, whereas amino acid PET may detect foci of a high-grade glioma within a lower grade tumor.[34] Contrast enhancement has been shown to be a strong predictor of malignancy. However, contrast enhancement may be missing in up to 10% of high-grade gliomas and up to 33% of anaplastic astrocytomas.[35,36] Moreover, a subset of low-grade tumors may present with contrast enhancement on MR imaging.[37] PET imaging might provide additional information to reveal the location of highest metabolic activity, and thus the aggressiveness of the tumor and the most appropriate site of biopsy. FDG-PET has been shown to be superior to MR imaging or CT alone for selecting the target displaying the highest tumoral grade.[38,39] However, these studies have not been limited to tumors without contrast enhancement, and the true and clinically relevant added value of PET cannot be definitively determined.

**A**

**B**

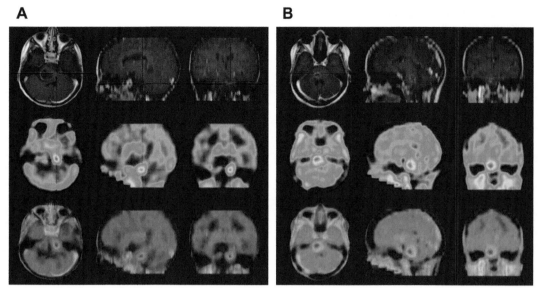

Fig. 1. Illustration of the difficulties to grade tumor from MR images alone and the potential aid provided by [18]F-fluoro-ethyl-L-tyrosine (FET) PET. (*A*) Brain lesion in a 4-year-old boy with high-grade tumor characteristics on MR imaging and spectroscopy (*top row*), [18]F-FET-PET (*middle row*), and PET–MR fusion (*bottom row*) images showing relatively high tumor-to-background ratio (TBR) = 1.8/0.8 = 2.3 but an early-to-middle (e-m) $SUV_{max}$ ratio of 0.73 indicating low-grade glioma (<0.90).[1] The final diagnosis was pilocytic astrocytoma (WHO grade I), as suggested by the [18]F-FET-PET. (*B*) Brain lesion in a 29-year-old woman with low-grade tumor characteristics on MR imaging and spectroscopy (*top row*), [18]F-FET-PET (*middle row*), and PET–MR fusion (*bottom row*) images showing relatively high TBR = 4.8/1.4 = 3.4 and an e-m ratio of 0.94 indicates high-grade glioma ($\geq$0.90).[1] The final diagnosis was glioblastoma (WHO grade IV), as supported by the [18]F-FET-PET result (see the article by Prior and colleagues elsewhere in this issue).

In one study of 81 patients, a discrepancy was noted in 38% of patients between the diagnosis made from biopsy samples and the final diagnosis established on the resected tumor specimen.[40] A recent report also suggests that FET-PET with a dynamic analysis may be able to detect anaplastic foci and differentiate between grade II and grade III histopathologies within one and the same lesion (sensitivity 92%, specificity 82%).[34]

To determine tumor sites with the highest grade, multimodality approaches showing contrast enhancement on T1-weighted MR imaging, a high choline peak on MR spectroscopy, and hypermetabolism on FET-PET or MET-PET may be warranted.[41] Two separate studies demonstrated the superiority in diagnostic accuracy (in this case, showing a higher tumor grade) of PET–MR fusion to guide diagnostic biopsy compared with MR imaging alone in gliomas without MR imaging contrast enhancement,[42,43] with increased specificity from about 50% for MR alone to more than 90% for PET–MRI fusion.

## PLANNING OF SURGERY: DEFINITION OF TUMOR EXTENT AND DELINEATION

Delineation of the margins and extent of the tumor by standard MR imaging alone lacks precision.

This lack of precision is not only because of the infiltrative nature of glioma but also because of the presence of edema or scar tissue and changes resulting from previous surgery or radiation therapy. Maximal and complete surgery have been shown to be a prognostic factor for progression-free and overall survival in both low-grade and high-grade gliomas, so that metabolic identification of tumor tissue may lead to a more extensive resection.[44] To date, only 2 uncontrolled studies have included PET evaluation in the planning of neurosurgical resection. Both studies have concluded that the incorporation of amino acid PET imaging resulted in an increased number of complete resections, which was associated with extended survival.[45]

## DIFFERENTIATION OF TUMOR RECURRENCE FROM TREATMENT EFFECTS

An accurate and early assessment of response to treatment is indispensable for the correct management of patients.[46] Such assessment prevents prolonged use of a potentially toxic and ineffective therapeutic agent and allows for rapidly changing to a more appropriate treatment strategy. However, the differentiation between residual tumor or tumor recurrence and posttherapeutic scar tissue may be challenging (**Box 2**).

The currently available limited data on FDG-PET are inconsistent and show only limited accuracy to reliably differentiate between treatment-induced necrosis and tumor with sensitivities and specificities between 40% and 90%.[17,58–60] Because radiolabeled amino acids are not metabolized by glycolytic inflammatory cells, they might be more appropriate markers to differentiate between recurrence of disease and nonspecific treatment-related changes. Several small studies have suggested that MET-PET (sensitivity, 75%–90%; specificity, 75%–92%) or FET-PET (positive predictive value, 84%; sensitivity, 82%; specificity, 100%) may increase the diagnostic accuracy.[61–65]

## PET AS A PROGNOSTIC TOOL

Despite numerous histologic (tumor grade), molecular (Ki1-67 proliferation index, epidermal growth factor receptor overexpression, *MGMT* promoter methylation, and others), and clinical (age, performance status, extent of resection) prognostic factors and markers, establishing a patient's individual prognosis remains highly difficult.[66] Some investigators suggested that FDG-PET might be used as a prognostic marker for patients with gliomas.[12,66–69] As an example, in high-grade gliomas the ratio of FDG-PET uptake between the tumor and the controlateral side was shown to predict the overall survival independent of other known prognostic factors such as age, performance status, histologic grade, and extent of surgery in a small retrospective study of 41

---

**Box 2**
**Radiation necrosis, imaging, and pseudoprogression**

Differentiation between radiation-induced or radiochemotherapy-induced necrosis, pseudoprogression, and true recurrence of tumor is of great importance and clinical relevance. With the combination of radiation therapy and temozolomide, an increased occurrence of treatment-induced necrosis (often termed as pseudoprogression) has been described in up to 45% of patients.[47] Pseudoprogression can be observed several weeks after the end of radiotherapy but may also occur as late as 3 to 6 months after the end of treatment. On MR imaging, all these changes may result in similar abnormal contrast enhancement. Moreover, conventional MR imaging techniques usually fail to detect early effects of radiotherapy or chemotherapy.[48,49] This failure results in significant interobserver variability in the evaluation of treatment response.[50] The definitive diagnosis of pseudoprogression can only be established retrospectively based on the spontaneously favorable outcome. In a series of patients operated shortly after the end of radiochemotherapy for presumed tumor progression, up to 50% of the samples did not contain any viable tumor cells. Interpretation may be further complicated by the presence of both necrosis and pseudoprogression and residual active tumor within the same MR imaging location.[51] Patients with methylated O-6methylguanine-DNA methyltransferase (*MGMT*) promoter present pseudoprogession more frequently, presumably because of a higher responsiveness to treatment.[52]

The combination of radiation therapy and chemotherapy results in increased risk of radiation toxicity.[53] The following 3 major types of radiation injury are distinguished:

- Acute injury occurs hours to weeks after radiation therapy and involves tumor swelling. Such is usually reversible and shows a good prognosis.
- Early delayed injury occurs weeks to months after completion of radiation therapy and involves reversible demyelination.
- Late injury is usually irreversible, occurring months to years after radiation therapy and involves liquefactive or coagulation necrosis.

Radiation necrosis is characterized by disruption of the BBB, edema, and mass effect.[54] The pattern of radiation injury may vary from diffuse periventricular white matter lesions to focal or multifocal lesions with necrotic foci, hypocellular edges, and hyalinized blood vessels.[55] Patients may be asymptomatic or present symptoms of progressive focal neurologic deficits or raised intracranial pressure.[56] Treatment of radiation necrosis includes the use of steroids and bevacizumab.[57] Traditionally used hyperbaric oxygen has been shown to be of little use in this setting. On MR imaging, radionecrosis typically appears as a contrast-enhancing lesion. Perfusion and diffusion MR imaging show low regional blood flow with a high lactate or lipid peak. MR spectroscopy shows low choline with a high lactate or lipid peak. Low tracer uptake on single-photon emission CT and PET scans further enhances the suspicion of radionecrosis. The sensitivity and specificity of these features is, however, limited, and radiation necrosis may be difficult to differentiate from tumor growth.[54]

patients.[70] Recently, a study of 102 patients with grade II and III oligodendroglial tumors evaluated with MET-PET suggested that patients with prognostically more favorable 1p/19q codeleted tumors show an increased tumor–normal tissue uptake ratio than tumors without 1p/19q loss of heterozygosity.[71] No explanation for this counterintuitive observation was provided. In low-grade gliomas, the use of amino acid PET imaging for grading tumors based on uptake only has given controversial results, probably because there is an overlap in the tracer uptake between different grades, not all amino acids are transported using the same molecular mechanisms, and even low-grade gliomas may show increased tracer uptake with time.[72–77] Better results can be achieved when studying the uptake of the labeled amino acid into the tumor with time.[78]

All studies evaluating the prognostic value of PET, however, have included too small a number of patients to allow for multivariate analyses. Low MET-PET uptake was found to be a weak independent factor for better prognosis in a population of 47 patients with grade II, III, or IV tumors,[79] although the exact selection criteria for the patients enrolled in this retrospective study were poorly defined.

Chen and colleagues[80] evaluated the prognostic value of FLT-PET to determine the outcome of patients with recurrent high-grade gliomas. FLT uptake correlated with the proliferation index Ki-67 and appeared more reliable than FDG uptake. The investigators correlated an extended survival in patients showing reduced FLT uptake.

## MONITORING OF TUMOR RESPONSE BY PET

Being able to correctly assess the response to treatment is a key element in the management of patients with brain tumors. The current standard requires monitoring of the tumor by repetitive MR imaging. This approach requires that a sufficient amount of time elapses between 2 examinations to detect tumor growth or shrinkage. In high-grade glioma, the interval is usually 2 to 3 months; in low-grade glioma, it takes 6 to 12 months to detect significant morphologic changes. This duration may expose the patient for unnecessarily long periods to potentially ineffective therapy or may lead one to abandon valuable and active treatment precociously. It would be of great value to predict shortly after initiating a treatment whether a given therapeutic agent holds its promise and controls the tumor. Several studies have assessed the predictive value of PET in assessing response in high-grade gliomas and have suggested that this approach might provide additional information to the standard use of MR imaging.[81,82] Chen and colleagues[81] evaluated the predictive value of FLT-PET to determine the treatment response in 30 patients with recurrent high-grade gliomas treated with bevacizumab and irinotecan. FLT-PET scans were performed at baseline before starting treatment and then at 2 and 6 weeks after onset of therapy. Decreased uptake on FLT-PET scan as early as 2 weeks after starting treatment was significant in predicting a longer survival, but changes on FLT-PET at 6 weeks of treatment was the strongest predictor of overall survival and progression-free survival. This correlation was interesting, but needs confirmation in a study with a larger number of patients.

In a series of 25 patients with glioblastoma multiforme, a decrease in uptake of FET 1 to 2 weeks after completion of radiochemotherapy in comparison to pretreatment baseline evaluation was correlated with a better outcome.[83]

Another series of 11 patients with recurrent high-grade glioma undergoing bevacizumab treatment was evaluated with FET-PET and MR imaging. In the 5 patients who showed discordant results between MR imaging and PET, the evolution of the patient showed that the FET-PET was able to predict failure of treatment before the MR imaging examination.[84] The power of this study is however limited by its retrospective nature and the small sample size. In patients with recurrent high-grade gliomas treated with the antiangiogenic agent bevacizumab, high pretreatment FDG-PET uptake or a high tumor to contralateral control ratio was able to independently predict a poor response and outcome in a retrospective series of 25 patients.[85]

## WHAT ARE THE NEXT STEPS FOR PET IMAGING IN NEURO-ONCOLOGY

Most PET imaging studies have mainly focused on the technical aspects of the methodology and have attempted to demonstrate equivalence or superiority to standard imaging or correlation and prediction of pathologic tumor grade. Some benefit of PET was suggested for the differentiation between treatment effect and tumor recurrence, exact localization and determination of the optimal site of biopsy, or early response prediction. Nuclear medicine societies have established guidelines and indications for the use of this diagnostic modality with FDG-PET[86] and amino acid PET,[87] as (summarized in **Table 2**).

Most PET studies conducted so far in neuro-oncology are limited by the inclusion of a small number of patients, the absence of validation, as well as poorly defined and heterogeneous inclusion criteria. Studies were commonly conducted

**Table 2**
**Recommendations of specialized societies for the use of PET and PET/CT**

| | Tracer: FDG | | |
| --- | --- | --- | --- |
| Indication | German Society for Nuklearmedizin (DGN), 2001[92] | Swiss Society for Nuclear Medicine (SGNM), 2008 | American College of Radiology (ACR), 2007 |
| Differentiation between recurrence and radiation necrosis | Recommended | Recommended | Recommended |
| Identification of malignant dedifferentiation of recurrent low-grade tumor | Recommended | Recommended | Recommended |
| Determination of biopsy site in gliomas | Recommended | Recommended | Recommended |
| Determination of biologic aggressiveness of tumor | Recommended | Recommended | Recommended |
| Determination of residual tumor after surgery | Recommended | Recommended | Recommended |
| | Tracer: Amino Acids | | |
| Indication | European Association of Nuclear Medicine (EANM), 2006 | | German Society for Nuklearmedizin (DGN) 2011[46] |
| Differentiation between recurrence and radiation necrosis | Recommended | | Recommended |

in single highly specialized centers and were often retrospective in nature. This limitation was especially highlighted by the German Institute for Quality in Health Care that conducted an in-depth review of the role of PET and PET-CT for the diagnosis of recurrences in high-grade gliomas[88] but applies similarly for other indications in neuro-oncology.

The question to date is therefore not what could be achieved by PET imaging in large multicentric studies as compared with a gold standard, but rather why PET imaging has not yet been able to obtain an established position for the management of these patients and why is it not used more systematically? One possible answer to this discrepancy is that studies in the field have focused mainly on demonstrating the feasibility of the techniques for a given clinical question. Only a few studies have actually addressed in a prospective manner the specificity and sensitivity of the PET technique as compared with available gold standards. Rather than comparing competing imaging techniques, we need to establish imaging protocols combining the rational and economical use of the different technologies available to be able to answer specific clinical questions. Ideally, it should be demonstrated that this approach results in a modification of patient management and in improved outcome (eg,

prolonged survival, less toxicity or shorter exposure to ineffective therapy, reduced use of resources). Ultimately, the impact of these novel techniques on drug development (early, more accurate response assessment), treatment morbidity, quality of life, and survival needs to be demonstrated. Appropriate and ideally randomized clinical trials need to be designed, which will ensure that PET-based imaging will benefit patients when indicated, rather than the current fairly individualized and resource-driven use of PET scan. These studies, however, will require several years. Moreover, the high-cost radiotracers and the absence of patent protection further impedes the realization of such studies. As a solution to overcome these difficulties, the tracer compounds used in PET imaging should obtain orphan drugs status for CNS cancers with eased approval and reimbursement. Obligation to enroll patients in prospective studies or at least to establish registries and surveillance of patient outcomes is needed to move the field forward. The technology seems to be highly valuable and useful; however, indications and impact in clinical management need to be documented and validated. This will allow to demonstrate efficacy and impact in patient outcome. The feasibility and value of this approach has already been demonstrated with the National Oncologic PET registry

(NOPR) in the United States for a large number of indications in oncology and could easily be adapted to specific neuro-oncology questions.[89–91]

## REFERENCES

1. Hottinger AF, Stupp R. Therapeutic strategies for the management of gliomas. Rev Neurol (Paris) 2008; 164:523–30 [Article in French].
2. Stupp R, Hottinger AF, van den Bent MJ, et al. Frequently asked questions in the medical management of high-grade glioma: a short guide with practical answers. Ann Oncol 2008;19(Suppl 7): vii209–16.
3. Horska A, Barker PB. Imaging of brain tumors: MR spectroscopy and metabolic imaging. Neuroimaging Clin N Am 2010;20:293–310.
4. Del Sole A, Falini A, Ravasi L, et al. Anatomical and biochemical investigation of primary brain tumours. Eur J Nucl Med 2001;28:1851–72.
5. Levivier M, Becerra A, De Witte O, et al. Radiation necrosis or recurrence. J Neurosurg 1996;84:148–9.
6. Herholz K, Wienhard K, Heiss WD. Validity of PET studies in brain tumors. Cerebrovasc Brain Metab Rev 1990;2:240–65.
7. Gambhir SS. Molecular imaging of cancer with positron emission tomography. Nat Rev Cancer 2002;2: 683–93.
8. Jacobs AH, Dittmar C, Winkeler A, et al. Molecular imaging of gliomas. Mol Imaging 2002;1:309–35.
9. Phelps ME, Coleman RE. Nuclear medicine in the new millennium. J Nucl Med 2000;41:1–4.
10. Roelcke U. Imaging brain tumors with PET, SPECT, and ultrasonography. Handb Clin Neurol 2012;104: 135–42.
11. Wong TZ, van der Westhuizen GJ, Coleman RE. Positron emission tomography imaging of brain tumors. Neuroimaging Clin N Am 2002;12:615–26.
12. Padma MV, Said S, Jacobs M, et al. Prediction of pathology and survival by FDG PET in gliomas. J Neurooncol 2003;64:227–37.
13. Patronas NJ, Di Chiro G, Brooks RA, et al. Work in progress: [18F] fluorodeoxyglucose and positron emission tomography in the evaluation of radiation necrosis of the brain. Radiology 1982;144:885–9.
14. Di Chiro G. Positron emission tomography using [18F] fluorodeoxyglucose in brain tumors. A powerful diagnostic and prognostic tool. Invest Radiol 1987;22:360–71.
15. Glantz MJ, Hoffman JM, Coleman RE, et al. Identification of early recurrence of primary central nervous system tumors by [18F]fluorodeoxyglucose positron emission tomography. Ann Neurol 1991;29:347–55.
16. Olivero WC, Dulebohn SC, Lister JR. The use of PET in evaluating patients with primary brain tumours: is it useful? J Neurol Neurosurg Psychiatry 1995;58: 250–2.
17. Ricci PE, Karis JP, Heiserman JE, et al. Differentiating recurrent tumor from radiation necrosis: time for re-evaluation of positron emission tomography? AJNR Am J Neuroradiol 1998;19:407–13.
18. Weber W, Bartenstein P, Gross MW, et al. Fluorine-18-FDG PET and iodine-123-IMT SPECT in the evaluation of brain tumors. J Nucl Med 1997;38:802–8.
19. Wong TZ, Turkington TG, Hawk TC, et al. PET and brain tumor image fusion. Cancer J 2004;10:234–42.
20. Pirotte B, Goldman S, Massager N, et al. Combined use of 18F-fluorodeoxyglucose and 11C-methionine in 45 positron emission tomography-guided stereotactic brain biopsies. J Neurosurg 2004;101:476–83.
21. Chen W, Silverman DH, Delaloye S, et al. 18F-FDOPA PET imaging of brain tumors: comparison study with 18F-FDG PET and evaluation of diagnostic accuracy. J Nucl Med 2006;47:904–11.
22. Laverman P, Boerman OC, Corstens FH, et al. Fluorinated amino acids for tumour imaging with positron emission tomography. Eur J Nucl Med Mol Imaging 2002;29:681–90.
23. Jager PL, Vaalburg W, Pruim J, et al. Radiolabeled amino acids: basic aspects and clinical applications in oncology. J Nucl Med 2001;42:432–45.
24. Miyagawa T, Oku T, Uehara H, et al. "Facilitated" amino acid transport is upregulated in brain tumors. J Cereb Blood Flow Metab 1998;18:500–9.
25. Sasajima T, Miyagawa T, Oku T, et al. Proliferation-dependent changes in amino acid transport and glucose metabolism in glioma cell lines. Eur J Nucl Med Mol Imaging 2004;31:1244–56.
26. Roelcke U, Radu EW, von Ammon K, et al. Alteration of blood-brain barrier in human brain tumors: comparison of [18F]fluorodeoxyglucose, [11C] methionine and rubidium-82 using PET. J Neurol Sci 1995;132:20–7.
27. Ishiwata K, Kubota K, Murakami M, et al. Re-evaluation of amino acid PET studies: can the protein synthesis rates in brain and tumor tissues be measured in vivo? J Nucl Med 1993;34:1936–43.
28. Weber WA, Wester HJ, Grosu AL, et al. O-(2-[18F]fluoroethyl)-L-tyrosine and L-[methyl-11C]methionine uptake in brain tumours: initial results of a comparative study. Eur J Nucl Med 2000;27:542–9.
29. Becherer A, Karanikas G, Szabo M, et al. Brain tumour imaging with PET: a comparison between [18F]fluorodopa and [11C]methionine. Eur J Nucl Med Mol Imaging 2003;30:1561–7.
30. Barwick T, Bencherif B, Mountz JM, et al. Molecular PET and PET/CT imaging of tumour cell proliferation using F-18 fluoro-L-thymidine: a comprehensive evaluation. Nucl Med Commun 2009;30:908–17.
31. Saga T, Kawashima H, Araki N, et al. Evaluation of primary brain tumors with FLT-PET: usefulness and limitations. Clin Nucl Med 2006;31:774–80.
32. Pichler R, Dunzinger A, Wurm G, et al. Is there a place for FET PET in the initial evaluation of brain

lesions with unknown significance? Eur J Nucl Med Mol Imaging 2010;37:1521–8.

33. Dunet V, Rossier C, Buck A, et al. Performance of 18F-fluoro-ethyl-tyrosine (18F-FET) PET for the differential diagnosis of primary brain tumor: a systematic review and metaanalysis. J Nucl Med 2012;53:207–14.

34. Kunz M, Thon N, Eigenbrod S, et al. Hot spots in dynamic (18)FET-PET delineate malignant tumor parts within suspected WHO grade II gliomas. Neuro Oncol 2011;13:307–16.

35. Scott JN, Brasher PM, Sevick RJ, et al. How often are nonenhancing supratentorial gliomas malignant? A population study. Neurology 2002;59:947–9.

36. Barker FG IInd, Chang SM, Huhn SL, et al. Age and the risk of anaplasia in magnetic resonance-nonenhancing supratentorial cerebral tumors. Cancer 1997;80:936–41.

37. Law M, Yang S, Wang H, et al. Glioma grading: sensitivity, specificity, and predictive values of perfusion MR imaging and proton MR spectroscopic imaging compared with conventional MR imaging. AJNR Am J Neuroradiol 2003;24:1989–98.

38. Pirotte BJ, Lubansu A, Massager N, et al. Results of positron emission tomography guidance and reassessment of the utility of and indications for stereotactic biopsy in children with infiltrative brainstem tumors. J Neurosurg 2007;107:392–9.

39. Pirotte BJ, Lubansu A, Massager N, et al. Clinical impact of integrating positron emission tomography during surgery in 85 children with brain tumors. J Neurosurg Pediatr 2010;5:486–99.

40. Jackson RJ, Fuller GN, Abi-Said D, et al. Limitations of stereotactic biopsy in the initial management of gliomas. Neuro Oncol 2001;3:193–200.

41. Goldman S, Levivier M, Pirotte B, et al. Regional glucose metabolism and histopathology of gliomas. A study based on positron emission tomography-guided stereotactic biopsy. Cancer 1996;78:1098–106.

42. Pauleit D, Floeth F, Hamacher K, et al. O-(2-[18F]fluoroethyl)-L-tyrosine PET combined with MRI improves the diagnostic assessment of cerebral gliomas. Brain 2005;128:678–87.

43. Floeth FW, Pauleit D, Wittsack HJ, et al. Multimodal metabolic imaging of cerebral gliomas: positron emission tomography with [18F]fluoroethyl-L-tyrosine and magnetic resonance spectroscopy. J Neurosurg 2005;102:318–27.

44. McGirt MJ, Chaichana KL, Gathinji M, et al. Independent association of extent of resection with survival in patients with malignant brain astrocytoma. J Neurosurg 2009;110:156–62.

45. Pirotte BJ, Levivier M, Goldman S, et al. Positron emission tomography-guided volumetric resection of supratentorial high-grade gliomas: a survival analysis in 66 consecutive patients. Neurosurgery 2009; 64:471–81.

46. Langen KJ, Bartenstein P, Boecker H, et al. German guidelines for brain tumour imaging by PET and SPECT using labelled amino acids. Nuklearmedizin 2011;50:167–73 [Article in German].

47. Chamberlain MC. Pseudoprogression in glioblastoma. J Clin Oncol 2008;26:4359.

48. Kumar AJ, Leeds NE, Fuller GN, et al. Malignant gliomas: MR imaging spectrum of radiation therapy- and chemotherapy-induced necrosis of the brain after treatment. Radiology 2000;217:377–84.

49. de Wit MC, de Bruin HG, Eijkenboom W, et al. Immediate post-radiotherapy changes in malignant glioma can mimic tumor progression. Neurology 2004;63:535–7.

50. Vos MJ, Uitdehaag BM, Barkhof F, et al. Interobserver variability in the radiological assessment of response to chemotherapy in glioma. Neurology 2003;60:826–30.

51. Chamberlain MC, Glantz MJ, Chalmers L, et al. Early necrosis following concurrent Temodar and radiotherapy in patients with glioblastoma. J Neurooncol 2007;82:81–3.

52. Brandes AA, Franceschi E, Tosoni A, et al. *MGMT* promoter methylation status can predict the incidence and outcome of pseudoprogression after concomitant radiochemotherapy in newly diagnosed glioblastoma patients. J Clin Oncol 2008;26: 2192–7.

53. Hustinx R, Pourdehnad M, Kaschten B, et al. PET imaging for differentiating recurrent brain tumor from radiation necrosis. Radiol Clin North Am 2005;43:35–47.

54. Alexiou GA, Tsiouris S, Kyritsis AP, et al. Glioma recurrence versus radiation necrosis: accuracy of current imaging modalities. J Neurooncol 2009;95: 1–11.

55. Perry A, Schmidt RE. Cancer therapy-associated CNS neuropathology: an update and review of the literature. Acta Neuropathol 2006;111:197–212.

56. Giglio P, Gilbert MR. Cerebral radiation necrosis. Neurologist 2003;9:180–8.

57. Benoit A, Ducray F, Cartalat-Carel S, et al. Favorable outcome with bevacizumab after poor outcome with steroids in a patient with temporal lobe and brainstem radiation necrosis. J Neurol 2011;258:328–9.

58. Langleben DD, Segall GM. PET in differentiation of recurrent brain tumor from radiation injury. J Nucl Med 2000;41:1861–7.

59. Chao ST, Suh JH, Raja S, et al. The sensitivity and specificity of FDG PET in distinguishing recurrent brain tumor from radionecrosis in patients treated with stereotactic radiosurgery. Int J Cancer 2001; 96:191–7.

60. Barker FG IInd, Chang SM, Valk PE, et al. 18-Fluorodeoxyglucose uptake and survival of patients with suspected recurrent malignant glioma. Cancer 1997;79:115–26.

61. Ullrich RT, Kracht L, Brunn A, et al. Methyl-L-11C-methionine PET as a diagnostic marker for malignant progression in patients with glioma. J Nucl Med 2009;50:1962–8.

62. Terakawa Y, Tsuyuguchi N, Iwai Y, et al. Diagnostic accuracy of 11C-methionine PET for differentiation of recurrent brain tumors from radiation necrosis after radiotherapy. J Nucl Med 2008;49:694–9.

63. Van Laere K, Ceyssens S, Van Calenbergh F, et al. Direct comparison of 18F-FDG and 11C-methionine PET in suspected recurrence of glioma: sensitivity, inter-observer variability and prognostic value. Eur J Nucl Med Mol Imaging 2005;32:39–51.

64. Mehrkens JH, Popperl G, Rachinger W, et al. The positive predictive value of O-(2-[18F]fluoroethyl)-L-tyrosine (FET) PET in the diagnosis of a glioma recurrence after multimodal treatment. J Neurooncol 2008; 88:27–35.

65. Popperl G, Gotz C, Rachinger W, et al. Value of O-(2-[18F]fluoroethyl)- L-tyrosine PET for the diagnosis of recurrent glioma. Eur J Nucl Med Mol Imaging 2004;31:1464–70.

66. Lote K, Egeland T, Hager B, et al. Survival, prognostic factors, and therapeutic efficacy in low-grade glioma: a retrospective study in 379 patients. J Clin Oncol 1997;15:3129–40.

67. Piepmeier J, Christopher S, Spencer D, et al. Variations in the natural history and survival of patients with supratentorial low-grade astrocytomas. Neurosurgery 1996;38:872–8.

68. Alavi JB, Alavi A, Chawluk J, et al. Positron emission tomography in patients with glioma. A predictor of prognosis. Cancer 1988;62:1074–8.

69. Patronas NJ, Di Chiro G, Kufta C, et al. Prediction of survival in glioma patients by means of positron emission tomography. J Neurosurg 1985;62:816–22.

70. Colavolpe C, Metellus P, Mancini J, et al. Independent prognostic value of pre-treatment 18-FDG-PET in high-grade gliomas. J Neurooncol 2012; 107:527–35.

71. Saito T, Maruyama T, Muragaki Y, et al. 11C-Methionine uptake correlates with combined 1p and 19q loss of heterozygosity in oligodendroglial tumors. AJNR Am J Neuroradiol 2012. in press.

72. Klasner BD, Krause BJ, Beer AJ, et al. PET imaging of gliomas using novel tracers: a sleeping beauty waiting to be kissed. Expert Rev Anticancer Ther 2010;10:609–13.

73. Okubo S, Zhen HN, Kawai N, et al. Correlation of L-methyl-11C-methionine (MET) uptake with L-type amino acid transporter 1 in human gliomas. J Neurooncol 2010;99:217–25.

74. Pauleit D, Stoffels G, Bachofner A, et al. Comparison of (18)F-FET and (18)F-FDG PET in brain tumors. Nucl Med Biol 2009;36:779–87.

75. Plotkin M, Blechschmidt C, Auf G, et al. Comparison of F-18 FET-PET with F-18 FDG-PET for biopsy planning of non-contrast-enhancing gliomas. Eur Radiol 2010;20:2496–502.

76. Herholz K, Holzer T, Bauer B, et al. 11C-methionine PET for differential diagnosis of low-grade gliomas. Neurology 1998;50:1316–22.

77. Fueger BJ, Czernin J, Cloughesy T, et al. Correlation of 6-18F-fluoro-L-dopa PET uptake with proliferation and tumor grade in newly diagnosed and recurrent gliomas. J Nucl Med 2010;51:1532–8.

78. Calcagni ML, Galli G, Giordano A, et al. Dynamic O-(2-[18F]fluoroethyl)-L-tyrosine (F-18 FET) PET for glioma grading: assessment of individual probability of malignancy. Clin Nucl Med 2011;36:841–7.

79. Kim S, Chung JK, Im SH, et al. 11C-methionine PET as a prognostic marker in patients with glioma: comparison with 18F-FDG PET. Eur J Nucl Med Mol Imaging 2005;32:52–9.

80. Chen W, Cloughesy TF, Kamdar N, et al. Imaging proliferation in brain tumors with 18F-FLT PET: comparison with 18F-FDG. J Nucl Med 2005;46:946–52.

81. Chen W, Delaloye S, Silverman DH, et al. Predicting treatment response of malignant gliomas to bevacizumab and irinotecan by imaging proliferation with [18F] fluorothymidine positron emission tomography: a pilot study. J Clin Oncol 2007;25:4714–21.

82. Schwarzenberg J, Czernin J, Cloughesy TF, et al. 3'-Deoxy-3'-18F-fluorothymidine PET and MRI for early survival predictions in patients with recurrent malignant glioma treated with bevacizumab. J Nucl Med 2012;53:29–36.

83. Holzer T, Herholz K, Jeske J, et al. FDG-PET as a prognostic indicator in radiochemotherapy of glioblastoma. J Comput Assist Tomogr 1993;17:681–7.

84. Hutterer M, Nowosielski M, Putzer D, et al. O-(2-18F-fluoroethyl)-L-tyrosine PET predicts failure of antiangiogenic treatment in patients with recurrent high-grade glioma. J Nucl Med 2011;52:856–64.

85. Colavolpe C, Chinot O, Metellus P, et al. FDG-PET predicts survival in recurrent high-grade gliomas treated with bevacizumab and irinotecan. Neuro Oncol 2012;14:649–57.

86. Varrone A, Asenbaum S, Vander Borght T, et al. EANM procedure guidelines for PET brain imaging using [18F]FDG, version 2. Eur J Nucl Med Mol Imaging 2009;36:2103–10.

87. Vander Borght T, Asenbaum S, Bartenstein P, et al. EANM procedure guidelines for brain tumour imaging using labelled amino acid analogues. Eur J Nucl Med Mol Imaging 2006;33:1374–80.

88. Gesundheitswesen I f Q u W i. D06–01D_Abschlussbericht_PET_und_PET-CT_bei_malignen_Gliomen. 2010.

89. Tunis S, Whicher D. The National Oncologic PET Registry: lessons learned for coverage with evidence development. J Am Coll Radiol 2009;6:360–5.

90. Hillner BE, Liu D, Coleman RE, et al. The national oncologic PET registry (NOPR): design and analysis plan. J Nucl Med 2007;48:1901–8.

91. Hillner BE, Siegel BA, Shields AF, et al. Impact of dedicated brain PET on intended patient management in participants of the national oncologic PET Registry. Mol Imaging Biol 2011;13: 161–5.

92. Reske SN, Kotzerke J. FDG-PET for clinical use. Results of the 3rd German interdisciplinary consensus conference, "Onko-PET III", 21 July and 19 September 2000. Eur J Nucl Med 2001;28: 1707–23.

# Overview of PET Tracers for Brain Tumor Imaging

Akash Sharma, MD[a], Jonathan McConathy, MD, PhD[a,b,*]

## KEYWORDS

- Brain tumors • Glioma • Radiotracers • Amino acids • $^{18}$F-Fluorodeoxyglucose
- $^{18}$F-Fluorothymidine

## KEY POINTS

- This article provides an overview of the key considerations for the development and application of molecular imaging agents for brain tumors, and the major classes of PET tracers that have been used for imaging brain tumors in humans.
- The most widely used PET tracers for this application are the glucose analogue 2-deoxy-2-[$^{18}$F]fluoro-D-glucose ($^{18}$F-FDG), radiolabeled amino acids (eg, $^{11}$C-MET, $^{18}$F-FET, $^{18}$F-FDOPA), and the nucleoside analogue 3′-deoxy-3′-fluorothymidine ($^{18}$F-FLT).
- Other PET tracers that have been evaluated in patients with brain tumor include hypoxia imaging agents, [$^{11}$C]choline, [$^{11}$C]acetate, and the $^{68}$Ga-labeled somatostatin receptor ligands DOTATOC and DOTATATE.
- The available data indicate that several of these classes of tracers, including radiolabeled amino acids, have imaging properties superior to those of $^{18}$F-FDG, and can complement contrast-enhanced magnetic resonance imaging for estimation of tumor volume, evaluation of nonenhancing gliomas, monitoring of response to therapy, and distinguishing recurrent tumors from treatment effects including radiation necrosis.

## INTRODUCTION

This article provides an overview of the key considerations for the development and application of molecular imaging agents for brain tumors, and the major classes of PET tracers that have been used for imaging brain tumors in humans. The most widely used PET tracers for this application are the glucose analogue 2-deoxy-2-[$^{18}$F]fluoro-D-glucose ($^{18}$F-FDG); radiolabeled amino acids (AAs), for example, L-[$^{11}$C]methionine ($^{11}$C-MET), O-(2-[$^{18}$F]fluoroethyl)-L-tyrosine ($^{18}$F-FET), and 6-[$^{18}$F]fluoro-3,4-dihydroxy-L-phenylalanine ($^{18}$F-FDOPA); and the nucleoside analogue 3′-deoxy-3′-fluorothymidine ($^{18}$F-FLT). Other PET tracers that may play a role in the evaluation of brain tumors are also discussed, and include hypoxia-sensitive agents (eg, α-([$^{18}$F]fluoromethyl)-2-nitro-1H-imidazole-1-ethanol [fluoromisonidazole, $^{18}$F-FMISO]; [$^{60/62/64}$Cu]copper(II) diacetyl-2,3-bis($N^4$-methyl-3-thiosemicarbazone) [$^{60/62/64}$Cu-ATSM]), [$^{11}$C]acetate ($^{11}$C-ACE), [$^{11}$C]choline ($^{11}$C-CHO), and tracers binding to somatostatin receptors (eg, [$^{68}$Ga]DOTATOC and [$^{68}$Ga]DOTATATE). Many of these tracers are discussed in greater depth in other articles elsewhere in this issue, and an overview of the biochemical properties and imaging characteristics are summarized here.

[a] Division of Nuclear Medicine, Mallinckrodt Institute of Radiology, 510 South Kingshighway Boulevard, Campus Box 8223, St Louis, MO 63110, USA; [b] Division of Radiological Sciences, Mallinckrodt Institute of Radiology, 510 South Kingshighway Boulevard, Campus Box 8223, St Louis, MO 63110, USA
* Corresponding author. Mallinckrodt Institute of Radiology, 510 South Kingshighway Boulevard, Campus Box 8223, St Louis, MO 63110.
E-mail address: mcconathyj@mir.wustl.edu

PET Clin 8 (2013) 129–146
http://dx.doi.org/10.1016/j.cpet.2013.02.001
1556-8598/13/$ – see front matter © 2013 Elsevier Inc. All rights reserved.

Neuroimaging plays a key role in the diagnosis, treatment planning, and follow-up of patients with primary and metastatic brain tumors. Although a tissue diagnosis is almost always obtained for the diagnosis of primary brain tumors, serial imaging is typically performed over the course of a patient's diagnostic evaluation and post-therapy course. Key diagnostic issues for primary brain tumors are summarized in **Box 1** and include accurate anatomic localization, tumor grading, definition of tumor extent and margins for presurgical planning, identification of optimal location for biopsy, determination of the presence or absence of involvement of critical structures such as speech and motor centers (eloquent cortex), early assessment of response to therapy, and differentiation of viable tumor from the effects of therapy. For PET tracers to be clinically useful and cost-effective, they must complement other currently available neuroimaging and diagnostic techniques to address 1 or more of these clinical questions.

At present, magnetic resonance (MR) imaging with gadolinium contrast agents is the primary modality for the routine clinical imaging of primary and metastatic brain tumors. MR provides high soft-tissue contrast and high-resolution anatomic images, and can provide functional information through perfusion-weighted and diffusion-weighted sequences.[1,2] Functional MR imaging using the blood oxygen level determination (BOLD) technique can also be used to localize speech and primary motor centers to help plan surgical resections. However, MR has limitations in evaluating nonenhancing gliomas and differentiating radiation necrosis from recurrent tumor, and provides primarily anatomic information in the routine clinical setting.

---

**Box 1**
**Goals of imaging in neuro-oncology**

Distinguishing tumor from nonneoplastic brain lesions

Tumor localization

Definition of tumor margins

Biopsy guidance

Assessment of tumor grade and aggressiveness

Identifying markers for prognosis and therapy

Evaluation of completeness of surgical resection

Monitoring response to chemotherapy and radiation

Distinguishing recurrent tumor from radiation necrosis

---

PET has been used for brain tumor imaging in both research and clinical settings for more than 3 decades. In the United States, the glucose analogue [18]F-FDG is the primary molecular imaging tracer used clinically for brain tumors. In clinical neuro-oncology, [18]F-FDG is used primarily to differentiate recurrent tumor from radiation necrosis. Although [18]F-FDG is useful for this indication, other PET tracers have superior imaging properties and provide biological information not available through [18]F-FDG PET or contrast-enhanced MR imaging alone. One of the major limitations in applying many of these tracers is the relatively small number of prospective, adequately powered studies demonstrating that incorporating PET into the diagnostic workup of patients with brain tumors positively affects management and outcomes.

## CLASSIFICATION OF BRAIN TUMORS

The applications of PET tracers for brain tumors depend on both the type of tumor and the clinical or research question being addressed. Brain tumors can be divided broadly into primary brain tumors, which arise from the brain itself, and metastatic brain tumors, which originate from primary cancers outside of the brain. PET tracer development and applications for brain tumors have mainly focused on primary brain tumors, although there are important roles for PET in metastatic disease as well. This section highlights the classification of brain tumors relevant to PET imaging. More in-depth information about brain tumor classification and management can be found in several recent review articles.[3–7]

Both primary and metastatic brain tumors can be classified as intra-axial, which are located within the brain parenchyma, or extra-axial, which are intracranial but not within in the brain parenchyma itself. The location, number, and distribution of intracranial lesions helps generate appropriate differential diagnoses and may influence the selection of therapy. Nonneoplastic lesions such as radiation necrosis, infectious/inflammatory processes, hematomas, and infarctions can mimic brain tumors on neuroimaging studies, and some of these entities are discussed in more detail for specific tracers.

Metastatic brain tumors are more common than primary brain tumors, and occur in approximately 9% to 17% of patients with cancer.[5] The most common primary cancers associated with brain metastases are lung cancer, breast cancer, and melanoma which account for approximately 67% to 80% of cases of brain metastases. Brain metastases are most often intra-axial, but extra-axial metastases do occur in locations such as the dural layer of the meninges that line the brain and spinal cord. Treatment options for brain metastases include chemotherapy, whole-brain radiation, stereotactic radiosurgery (SRS), and surgical resection.[8] PET imaging currently plays a relatively minor role in the initial evaluation of known brain metastases, although whole-body [18]F-FDG PET is sometimes used to determine the location of the primary tumor in cases of known or suspected metastases. In this scenario, PET imaging may identify higher yield or more accessible lesions outside the brain for biopsy to establish a tissue diagnosis. PET imaging for metastatic brain tumors is most useful for differentiating recurrent tumor from radiation necrosis, both of which typically present as enhancing masses on contrast-enhanced MR imaging. The combination of the increasing use of SRS for treating patients with 3 or fewer brain metastases and the increasing effectiveness of systemic chemotherapy has increased the frequency of radiation necrosis in neuro-oncology patients.

There are many types of primary brain tumors, but a few histologies predominate.[7,9] Primary brain tumors can be divided into extra-axial tumors (arising from nonneural tissue such as the meninges or the pituitary) and intra-axial tumors (arising from the glial or neuronal tissues). The access of drugs and imaging agents to extra-axial tumors is not limited by the blood-brain barrier (BBB), whereas intra-axial tumors have varying degrees of BBB integrity depending on tumor grade and histology. Primary brain tumors very rarely metastasize outside the central nervous system (CNS), but can spread through local extension and, less often, through dissemination through the cerebrospinal fluid.

Of the primary intra-axial brain tumors, gliomas are the most common histology in adults. Much of the PET tracer development and applications for brain tumor imaging have focused on brain gliomas. Gliomas can originate from neural stem cells, progenitor cells, or dedifferentiated neural cells within the brain, and are subdivided based on their histology (eg, astrocytoma, oligodendroglioma) and their histologic features. Gliomas are divided into grades I, II, III, and IV based on World Health Organization (WHO) criteria. Grades I and II gliomas are considered low grade, and grades III and IV are considered high grade. Tumor grade is a key factor in prognosis and treatment selection, although tumor grade alone does not provide a complete assessment of the biological aggressiveness of gliomas.

Low-grade gliomas typically grow slowly, and patients may survive for many years even if untreated. Over time, however, low-grade gliomas often transform into higher-grade gliomas, which are more aggressive and typically fatal. Surgery with or without radiation therapy may be curative for low-grade gliomas. The most common form of glioma in adults is glioblastoma (grade IV), which is highly aggressive and infiltrative; patients with glioblastomas have median survival times of approximately 8 to 13 months despite maximal therapy. Gliomas frequently recur after therapy, and neuroimaging plays a key role in detecting recurrence through either routine interval imaging after treatment or at the onset of new clinical symptoms. In children, low-grade gliomas are more common than high-grade gliomas, and medulloblastoma is the most common aggressive pediatric primary brain tumor.

Meningiomas are a common primary brain tumor, and the vast majority of meningiomas are extra-axial, most often arising from the meninges lining the outer surface of the brain. Most meningiomas are benign and relatively slow growing (WHO grade I), and many are detected incidentally by computed tomography (CT) and MR imaging studies performed for other indications. However, some meningiomas have atypical features (WHO grade II) or are anaplastic (WHO grade III), and can be locally aggressive, tend to recur, and may invade the brain parenchyma.

Primary CNS lymphoma is a relatively uncommon primary brain tumor that by definition is confined to the CNS.[6,10] Primary CNS lymphoma has been associated with immunocompromise such as AIDS, but can occur in the immunocompetent population as well. [18]F-FDG PET and other tracers have been applied to primary CNS lymphoma in 2 specific scenarios: differentiating brain involvement by lymphoma from cerebral infection (particularly in the immunocompromised), and distinguishing primary CNS lymphoma from system lymphoma with CNS involvement owing to differences in prognosis and therapy. These applications are discussed further in the sections on specific tracers.

## PET TRACERS FOR BRAIN TUMOR IMAGING
### General Considerations

A broad range of PET tracers has been developed for oncologic imaging, with different physiochemical properties, biological targets, and radionuclides. Of these, only a small subset has been evaluated for brain tumor imaging in humans. There are several characteristics desirable for PET imaging agents for brain tumors, summarized in **Box 2**. The choice of radionuclide is an important consideration for designing and using PET

Box 2

**Optimal properties of PET tracers for brain tumor imaging**

Radionuclide with half-life suitable for batch production and remote distribution

Half-life of radionuclide matched to tracer pharmacokinetics

Radionuclide with favorable PET imaging properties

Simple, reliable, and inexpensive radiosynthesis

No patient preparation needed

Rapid pharmacokinetics allowing short interval between tracer injection and PET imaging

Tracer accumulation in tumor and nonneoplastic tissues not negatively affected by concurrent therapies or medications

High tumor-to-background ratios

Crosses the BBB for visualization of nonenhancing regions in gliomas

Lack of interfering radiolabeled metabolite formation

Suitable for simple quantification techniques

Table 1
Properties of selected PET radionuclides

| Radionuclide | Half-Life | Mean Positron Energy (keV) | Positron Percentage |
|---|---|---|---|
| Carbon-11 | 20.4 min | 386 | 100 |
| Nitrogen-13 | 9.97 min | 492 | 100 |
| Fluorine-18 | 109.8 min | 250 | 97 |
| Copper-60 | 23.7 min | 970 | 93 |
| Copper-62 | 9.7 min | 1319 | 98 |
| Copper-64 | 12.7 h | 278 | 18 |
| Gallium-68 | 67.7 min | 830 | 89 |
| Bromine-76 | 16.2 h | 1180 | 55 |
| Yttrium-86 | 14.7 h | 660 | 32 |
| Zirconium-89 | 3.3 d | 396 | 23 |
| Iodine-124 | 4.2 d | 820 | 23 |

*Data from* Available at: http://www.nndc.bnl.gov/chart/. Accessed January 20, 2013.

tracers for brain tumor imaging. Many of these desirable characteristics are shared by PET tracers targeting tumors outside of the CNS, but the BBB and the effects of treatment on the BBB and normal brain are critical factors in brain tumor imaging, and are discussed in more depth.

A range of PET radionuclides has been used for labeling tracers for brain tumor imaging, and selected radionuclides and their properties are shown in **Table 1**. The kinetic energy of the emitted positron and the percentage of decay events giving rise to positrons differ between radionuclides and affect imaging properties. Higher positron kinetic energy leads to a longer path length between the emitting nucleus and the annihilation event, which decreases spatial resolution. Radionuclides that decay with lower fractions of positron emission have decay events that contribute to patient dose but do not contribute to the diagnostic image. Also, some radionuclides such as bromine-76, zirconium-89, and iodine-124 emit high-energy γ-rays, which must be corrected for during PET imaging reconstruction, contribute to patient and personnel dose, and are challenging to shield.

Carbon-11, nitrogen-13, and fluorine-18 are widely available through small medical cyclotrons, although of these radionuclides only fluorine-18 has a half-life long enough for batch productions

of large number of dosages and for remote distribution. The short half-life of carbon-11 limits the use of effective brain tumor imaging agents such as $^{11}$C-MET and $^{11}$C-CHO to facilities with cyclotrons and on-site production capabilities. Gallium-68 is available through the long-lived germanium-68 generator system, which has the potential for widespread availability. The other radionuclides shown in **Table 1** require more specialized production capabilities. The longer-lived radionuclides such as copper-64, zirconium-89, and iodine-124, as well as radiopharmaceuticals containing them, are suitable for remote distribution. The majority of PET tracers for brain tumor imaging have been labeled with carbon-11 and fluorine-18, although there are a few examples of tracers labeled with radiometals and other radiohalogens.

A special consideration in brain tumor imaging is the BBB. The BBB is a complex, biologically active structure composed of endothelial cells, pericytes, microglia, and astrocytes, which limits the entry of many compounds into the brain.[11] Most low-grade gliomas have intact BBBs and do not enhance with the administration of intravenous CT or MR contrast agents. Although high-grade gliomas often have impaired BBBs and enhance with contrast, some high-grade gliomas do not enhance, and even enhancing high-grade gliomas including glioblastomas often have nonenhancing regions. The BBB also prevents many molecular imaging agents from reaching nonenhancing regions of glioma, which limits their utility for visualizing and characterizing the entire tumor volume.

Some small molecules such as [18]F-FMISO can diffuse across the BBB, allowing access of the tracer to the entire tumor volume. Many of the PET tracers used for brain tumor imaging are substrates for biological transporters. In some cases, the transport mechanism itself is the primary imaging target, as in the case of radiolabeled AAs. Other tracers such as [18]F-FDG and [18]F-FLT require biological transport and are subsequently trapped by various mechanisms intracellularly. In the case of polar or charged molecules, the relevant transporters must be active at the luminal surface of the BBB for the tracers to reach tumor regions without disrupted BBBs. Metastatic brain tumors disrupt the BBB, and extra-axial primary brain tumors are located outside of the BBB. For this reason, molecular imaging agents used for imaging brain metastases and meningiomas typically do not have the same BBB limitations as gliomas. Although PET tracers with poor BBB penetration are typically not ideal for imaging gliomas when evaluation of the entire tumor volume is desired, they may still be of use in evaluating brain lesions with disrupted BBBs, as demonstrated by contrast enhancement on MR imaging. One advantage of tracers that do not cross the BBB is the potential for very high tumor-to-brain ratios through a combination of high uptake in tumor regions with disrupted BBB and exclusion from normal brain tissue.

Another important consideration in brain tumor imaging is the effect of therapy on imaging features of both the tumor and the adjacent brain structures. PET and other molecular imaging agents have great potential to complement MR imaging for both monitoring the response to therapy and evaluating for tumor recurrence after therapy. For example, treatment with the antiangiogenic therapy bevacizumab, a monoclonal antibody targeting vascular endothelial growth factor, can cause dramatic changes in tumor appearance.[12,13] Enhancement on MR imaging can resolve dramatically because of decreased permeability of the BBB, but this change is not specific and does not necessarily indicate that the tumor has responded to therapy. Radiation therapy is a common component of treatment for high-grade primary brain tumors and for metastatic lesions, but can also lead to diagnostic challenges. Radiation therapy can lead to radiation necrosis, which typically appears as a mass lesion on MR imaging and is not readily distinguished from recurrent tumor. Finally, monitoring of treatment response to chemotherapy and detection of recurrent disease in nonenhancing brain tumors with MR imaging can be challenging, owing to the slow and sometimes absent interval change in both effectively treated and progressive tumors.

## 2-Deoxy-2-Fluoro-D-Glucose

The glucose analogue [18]F-FDG is the most widely used PET tracer for clinical oncologic imaging. The cellular uptake of [18]F-FDG is mediated by cell membrane–associated transporter proteins, especially GLUT1 and GLUT3.[14] Once inside the cell, [18]F-FDG undergoes phosphorylation through hexokinase enzymes, which trap [18]F-FDG-6-phosphate inside the cell owing to the negative charge of the phosphate group. Because of the lack of a 2-hydroxy group, [18]F-FDG cannot undergo further metabolism via the glycolytic pathway. In some tissues, the action of glucose-6-phosphatase can remove the phosphate group, regenerating [18]F-FDG, which can then undergo transport out of the cell. This pathway is shown schematically in **Fig. 1**. Many neoplasms, including gliomas and metastatic brain tumors, have increased rates of glucose uptake and rates of glycolysis, even in the presence of adequate oxygen levels, to support oxidative phosphorylation (the Warburg effect), which leads to higher levels of [18]F-FDG accumulation in tumors relative to normal tissues.

[18]F-FDG has several useful properties for brain tumor imaging, as well as several important limitations. Glucose transport (GLUT1) is active at the normal BBB, which allows [18]F-FDG to reach the entire tumor volume.[15] The uptake of [18]F-FDG by brain tumors is not flow dependent and is typically irreversible over the time course of PET studies. The amount of [18]F-FDG uptake by gliomas is correlated with tumor grade and prognosis.[16,17] [18]F-FDG also usually has greater uptake in recurrent high-grade gliomas than in radiation necrosis, which can be used to distinguish recurrent tumor from the effects of radiation therapy. However, the normal brain also has high uptake of [18]F-FDG, which can decrease or obscure the visualization of brain tumors. In addition, inflammatory lesions including brain abscesses, granulomatous inflammation for both infectious and noninfectious causes, and normal brain parenchyma adjacent to subacute intraparenchymal hemorrhages can also have high uptake of [18]F-FDG, decreasing the specificity of [18]F-FDG in differentiating tumor from nonmalignant etiology.

The primary use of [18]F-FDG in current clinical neuro-oncology is for differentiating recurrent high-grade glioma or brain metastases from radiation necrosis, and for distinguishing CNS lymphoma from infectious processes in the brain. Because posttreatment radiation necrosis can be

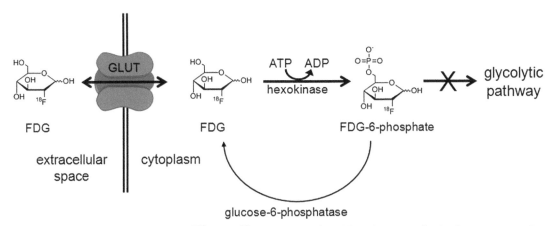

**Fig. 1.** Cellular uptake and trapping of [18]F-FDG. [18]F-FDG crosses the BBB and enters cells via glucose transporters (GLUTs) including GLUT1. Once in the cell, [18]F-FDG is trapped via phosphorylation by hexokinase enzymes. In some tissues, the enzyme glucose-6-phosphatase is active and can dephosphorylate [18]F-FDG-6-phosphate, allowing FDG to exit the cell via GLUTs. ADP, adenosine diphosphate; ATP, adenosine triphosphate.

variable in terms of morphology and progression, contrast-enhanced MR imaging alone has not been found to be reliable in this assessment. In the setting of changing or enlarging enhancing lesions, conventional MR imaging sequences are limited in the assessment of early recurrence.[18,19] [18]F-FDG imaging characteristics have been found to be more favorable than conventional (single-photon emission CT or SPECT) scintigraphy with thallium-201 in assessing brain lesions, especially when lesions were small.[20] In a typical patient, the higher resolution of PET, combined with the relatively hypometabolic background of the treated tumor bed, make it easier to assess for even small areas of hypermetabolism in the setting of early recurrence.[21] Furthermore, the ability to fuse [18]F-FDG PET images with various MR imaging sequences has been available for more than a decade, and has led to interest in studying the combined efficacy of [18]F-FDG with MR in assessing recurrent tumor versus radiation necrosis.

Although both MR imaging and [18]F-FDG PET are susceptible to false-positive outcomes for distinguishing radiation necrosis from recurrent tumor, the current clinical practice stresses the use of multiple MR sequences, including dynamic contrast-enhanced T1, diffusion-weighted imaging, and apparent diffusion coefficient sequences, in conjunction with [18]F-FDG PET images, to differentiate tumor recurrence from radiation necrosis. This combined approach shows promise and is an active area of investigation.[22,23] The differential kinetics of [18]F-FDG in radiation necrosis versus recurrent tumors have also been explored in hopes of increasing the diagnostic accuracy for this indication. A recent study with 32 subjects provides evidence that

dual time-point [18]F-FDG PET at approximately 1 hour and 3 to 6 hours after [18]F-FDG injection can more accurately distinguish recurrent brain metastases from treatment effects including radiation necrosis.[24] In this study, the sensitivity for recurrent tumor was high with both early and dual-phase imaging (89%–100%) when comparing uptake in the lesion with that in normal white matter, but the specificity increased substantially, from 67% with early imaging alone compared with 82% to 90% with dual time-point [18]F-FDG PET.

Semiquantitative assessment of FDG has been investigated in differentiating tumor recurrence from nonmalignant or benign processes and for targeted clinical issues such as lymphoma versus toxoplasmosis in immunocompromised patients. In few small studies, sensitivity and specificity for identifying lymphoma in the brain approached 74% to 100%, depending on whether a cutoff standardized uptake value (SUV) or a ratio of lesion to contralateral normal brain was used as the basis.[25,26] The infectious/nonlymphomatous lesions were identified by virtue of central hypometabolism in the setting of an enhancing lesion. As such, sensitivity and specificity were not directly calculated for such lesions. It is important to consider, however, that the ideal situation of lymphoma being discretely more intense than toxoplasmosis is not common, and significant variability of uptake is seen in both instances, leading to lower diagnostic accuracy in clinical practice.

## 3'-Deoxy-3'-Fluorothymidine

Nucleoside analogues have been used in a wide range of cancers for imaging the rate of proliferation of tumor cells. The accumulation of these tracers in tumor cells relies on the upregulation of DNA synthetic pathways, an indicator of increased cellular proliferation, in comparison with the normal brain cells. [18]F-FLT is a pyrimidine analogue of the naturally occurring nucleoside thymidine. The cellular uptake of [18]F-FLT occurs through a combination of passive diffusion and facilitated transport by type 1 equilibrative nucleoside transporters (ENT1).[27,28] Inside the cell, cytoplasmic thymidine kinase 1 (TK1) phosphorylates [18]F-FLT to [18]F-FLT-5-phosphate.[29] This pathway is shown schematically in **Fig. 2**. There may be upregulation of TK1 expression inside tumor or other rapidly proliferating cells, thus trapping [18]F-FLT in a greater proportion to normal brain cells. It has been established that [18]F-FLT does not undergo incorporation into DNA, and [18]F-FLT serves primarily as a marker of the fraction of tumor cells in the S-phase of cell cycle at the time of imaging (proliferation rate).[30] Other nucleoside analogues that undergo incorporation into DNA have been developed, including 1-(2′-deoxy-2′-[[18]F]fluoro-β-D-arabinofuranosyl)thymine (FMAU), but their utility in human brain tumor imaging remains to be established.

The whole-body biodistribution of [18]F-FLT is remarkable for greatest accumulation in the marrow, with additional relatively higher concentrations in liver and spleen, and excretion via the genitourinary system.[31] Unlike [18]F-FDG, [18]F-FLT does not readily cross the BBB, leading to very low uptake in normal brain. The cellular uptake of [18]F-FLT is also not specific to tumor cells, and any proliferative process may show increased [18]F-FLT uptake. Although the tumor cells may have relatively faster cell cycles with a greater fraction in the S-phase, there is still considerable variability of [18]F-FLT uptake within different tumors. The lower normal brain uptake of [18]F-FLT compared to [18]F-FDG may be an advantage for measuring proliferation rates in primary and metastatic brain tumors with disrupted BBBs.

With respect to primary intra-axial tumors of the brain, there is a high correlation between [18]F-FLT uptake as determined by semiquantitative analysis in the high-grade gliomas, whereas significant variability is present in terms of uptake in low-grade gliomas. In a study of 26 patients with untreated high-grade glioma, higher proliferative volumes of glioma tissue measured with [18]F-FLT PET were associated with poorer overall survival.[32]

In early comparison of [18]F-FLT with the more established [18]F-FDG evaluation for recurrent glioma, [18]F-FLT was shown to be more sensitive.[33] The absolute uptake of [18]F-FLT was much lower than for [18]F-FDG, but the tumor to normal brain ratios were higher. The utility of [18]F-FLT PET for measuring proliferation is supported by the positive correlation between uptake ($SUV_{max}$) and Ki-67 immunohistochemical measures of cell proliferation.[33–35] There are data suggesting that [18]F-FLT PET can serve as an early predictor for response to therapy in high-grade gliomas.[36] However, in comparing [18]F-FLT with other radiotracers under investigation, tracers including [18]F-FDOPA appear to be more accurate, especially when imaging lower-grade gliomas.[37,38]

As mentioned earlier, [18]F-FLT has been studied in whole-body distribution. In this context, it showed promising results in detecting lymphoma in the mediastinum, and it was posited that it may also be useful to evaluate lymphomatous

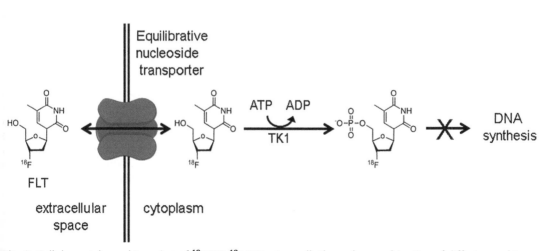

**Fig. 2.** Cellular uptake and trapping of [18]F-FLT. [18]F-FLT enters cells through a combination of diffusion and transport by the equilibrative nucleoside transporter 1 (ENT-1). Phosphorylation of [18]F-FLT is mediated by thymidine kinase 1 (TK1) and traps [18]F-FLT-5-phosphate within the cell, which cannot participate in DNA synthesis.

involvement of the brain.[31,39] However, in limited investigations the results are variable, and the most common outcome is that [18]F-FLT cannot reliably distinguish between tumors nor differentiate them from proliferating nontumorous lesions.

## Radiolabeled Amino Acids

AAs constitute a large class of structurally and biologically diverse small molecules that play vital roles in many cellular processes, including protein synthesis, energy metabolism, cell signaling, carbon sources for cell growth, and neurotransmission. AAs enter cells though membrane-associated proteins that vary greatly in their substrate specificity, tissue distribution, and biological properties.[40] In oncologic imaging applications, radiolabeled AAs target the higher rates of AA transport that occur in many tumor cells in comparison with many normal tissues. Although some radiolabeled AAs are incorporated into proteins or have other metabolic fates, tumor uptake and imaging properties primarily reflect the rate and mechanism of transport of the AA in most instances.[40,41]

AA transporters are membrane-associated proteins coded by family members of the solute carrier (SLC) series of genes that mediate the transfer of AAs across cell membranes. AA transporter families have traditionally been characterized functionally as transport systems (eg, system L, system A, system N, system ASC, system xCT), many of which contain multiple family members.[42–47] More than 20 distinct AA transport systems have been identified with different substrate specificities, tissue expression patterns, dependence on cotransport of ions such as sodium, hormonal regulation, mechanisms of transport, and biological significance in cancer.

There are numerous studies showing that certain radiolabeled AAs complement contrast-enhanced MR imaging for the evaluation of primary brain tumors. Virtually all of the currently available clinically useful radiolabeled AAs for brain tumor imaging are substrates for the system L family of AA transporters. System L consists of 4 family members coded for by SLC genes: LAT1 (SLC7A5), LAT2 (SLC7A8), LAT3 (SLC43A1), and LAT4 (SLC43A2). LAT1 is active at the BBB, allowing visualization of nonenhancing gliomas.[48] In addition, LAT1 is upregulated in many human cancers including gliomas, and higher levels of LAT1 are correlated with poorer survival.[49–51] The kinetics of AA uptake are relatively rapid, with peak tumor uptake typically occurring within 15 to 20 minutes of tracer injection.

System L transporters preferentially recognize AAs with large, neutral side chains, including L-phenylalanine, L-tyrosine, and L-leucine. LAT1 and LAT2 form functional heterodimers with the glycoprotein 4Fhc and mediate AA transport through a sodium-independent exchange mechanism, which leads to the import of an extracellular AA into the cell coupled with the export of an intracellular AA out of the cell in a 1:1 stoichiometry. LAT3 and LAT4 mediate AA transport through a facilitated diffusion mechanism that is also sodium independent. System L is not capable of directly concentrating its substrates intracellularly because of its mechanism of transport, limiting the tumor-to-brain ratios that can be achieved to no more than approximately 4:1.

The AAs that have been most used for PET imaging of brain tumors in humans are L-[11]C-MET, [18]F-FET, and [18]F-FDOPA.[52–54] The structures and mechanisms of uptake of these tracers are shown schematically in **Fig. 3**. The primary determinant of their tumor imaging properties seems to be rates of AA transporter rather than incorporation into proteins or involvement in other metabolic pathways. [18]F-FET is metabolically inert, whereas [11]C-MET and [18]F-FDOPA both undergo extensive intracellular metabolism. The lack of formation of radiolabeled metabolites may facilitate kinetic analysis of AA PET. [18]F-FDOPA has been used extensively for the evaluation of the central dopaminergic system as it is taken up and metabolized into 6-[[18]F]fluorodopamine, which is packaged into synaptic vesicles in dopaminergic nerve terminals. To a first approximation, [11]C-MET, [18]F-FET, and [18]F-FDOPA and other system L substrates have similar imaging properties in brain tumors.[55]

Radiolabeled AAs have been used for a wide range of applications for gliomas and metastatic brain tumors. For almost all neuro-oncology applications, radiolabeled AAs are clearly superior to [18]F-FDG PET. There are substantial data in brain gliomas demonstrating that [11]C-MET and [18]F-FET provide more accurate estimates of gross tumor volume and margins[56,57] and guidance for tumor biopsies[57–59] than contrast-enhanced MR imaging alone. There is also evidence that the kinetics of [18]F-FET can distinguish high-grade from low-grade gliomas, although this application requires further validation.[60–62] [11]C-MET, [18]F-FET, and [18]F-FDOPA have also been used to monitor response to therapy in nonenhancing gliomas, and can detect favorable response and recurrence earlier than MR imaging.[37,63,64] There are emerging data that [11]C-MET and [18]F-FET can distinguish recurrent tumor from radiation necrosis in brain metastases treated with SRS,[53,65–67]

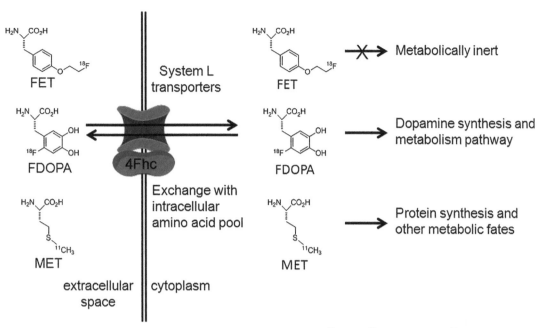

**Fig. 3.** Cellular uptake of the system AA transporter substrates [18]F-FET, [18]F-FDOPA, and [11]C-MET. System L substrates cross the BBB and enter cells through system L transporters that can mediate both AA uptake and efflux. Transport via LAT1 and LAT2 requires heterodimerization with the heavy-chain glycoprotein 4FHc (SLC3A2), and the mechanism of transport involves the exchange of an extracellular AA substrate with an intra-cellular AA. LAT3 and LAT4 mediate facilitated diffusion and do not require 4FHc. Once inside the cell, [18]F-FDOPA and [11]C-MET undergo further metabolism while [18]F-FET does not.

but more studies are needed to assess their accu-racy for this indication in a clinical setting.

There has been relatively little evaluation of ra-diolabeled AAs targeting other transport systems for brain tumor imaging in humans. One of the important potential limitations of tracers that are not substrates for system L transporters is the lack of activity of these AA transporters at the BBB. For example, the tracer cis-4-[18F]fluoro-L-proline (FPro) is transported by system A, which is not active at the luminal surface of the BBB.[68,69] Unlike system L tracers, the brain and tumor distribution of FPro was very similar to that of gadolinium MR contrast, suggesting that this tracer is not suitable for reliably delineating the non-enhancing regions within gliomas. Several AA PET agents targeting system A,[70–72] glutamine trans-port,[73,74] xCT transport,[70–72,75,76] and cationic AA transporters[77] have shown promising properties for brain tumor imaging in preclinical models, but their utility and roles for clinical imaging in neuro-oncology patients is not yet defined.

## HYPOXIA IMAGING

There are several PET tracers that accumulate in hypoxic regions of tumors,[78,79] and both [18]F-

FMISO and [60/62/64]Cu-ATSM have been used to image gliomas. Both tracers enter tumor cells through passive diffusion across cell membranes and become trapped intracellularly in hypoxic cells through reduction, as shown schematically in **Fig. 4.** Hypoxia is a common feature of many cancers including glioblastoma, due in part to tumors outgrowing their blood supply. Hypoxia is associated with tumor aggressiveness and resis-tance to radiotherapy and other treatments, and accurate identification of hypoxic regions within tumors has the potential to alter treatment plans. Both [18]F-FMISO and Cu-ATSM cross the BBB, although rigorous evaluation of their ability to eval-uate nonenhancing regions in gliomas has not been performed.

[18]F-FMISO PET studies have shown higher uptake in high-grade gliomas (particularly glioblas-tomas) than low-grade gliomas, and the tracer signal is typically located at the periphery of tumors in viable, hypoxic cells.[80–82] However, it is unclear whether tumor grading with [18]F-FMISO will be accurate enough for clinical decision making on an individual patient basis. Other studies have shown that higher uptake of [18]F-FMISO correlates with higher levels of angiogen-esis and higher proliferation rates, suggesting

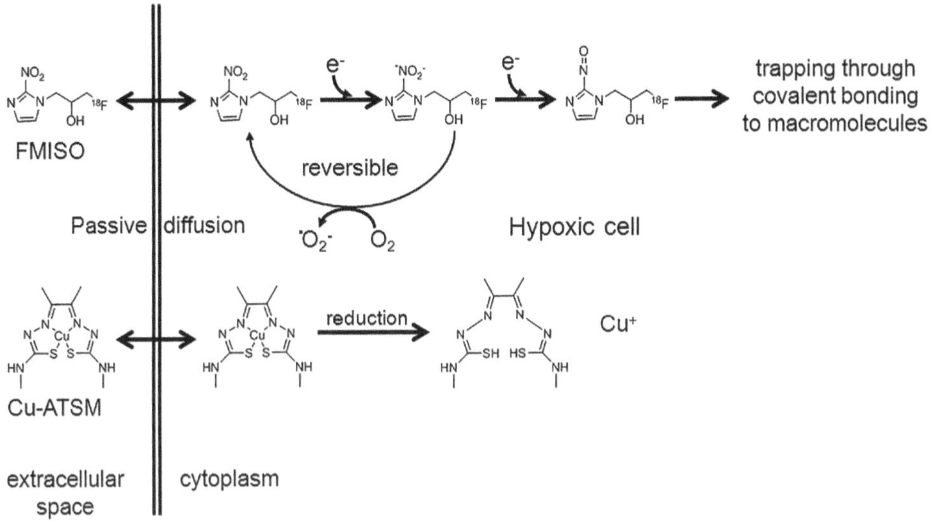

Fig. 4. Cellular uptake and trapping of $^{18}$F-FMISO and Cu-ATSM. The hypoxia-sensitive tracers $^{18}$F-FMISO and Cu-ATSM cross the BBB and enter cells via passive diffusion. In hypoxic cells, both tracers are reduced, which leads to retention inside cells through reaction with macromolecules in the case of $^{18}$F-FMISO and loss of copper in the case of Cu-ATSM.

that higher uptake corresponds to more aggressive tumors.[83,84]

There have been very few published studies with Cu-ATSM in brain tumors, but theoretical advantages of Cu-ATSM are higher signal to background ratios, faster pharmacokinetics allowing imaging earlier after injection than $^{18}$F-FMISO (approximate 30 minutes after injection compared with 2–4 hours for FMISO), and the flexibility of the different short and long half-lives of the radioisotopes of copper suitable for PET. A recent study evaluating the uptake of $^{62}$Cu-ATSM in gliomas demonstrated higher uptake in glioblastomas than in lower-grade gliomas,[85] similar to results reported for $^{18}$F-FMISO. The uptake of $^{62}$Cu-ATSM in this study also correlated with higher levels of hypoxia-induced factor 1α (HIF-1α), a marker of cellular hypoxia. The utility of $^{18}$F-FMISO and Cu-labeled ATSM for selecting the most appropriate treatment plan or improving patient outcomes has yet to be established.

## Choline and Fluorocholine

The PET tracers $^{11}$C-CHO and [$^{18}$F]fluorocholine (N,N-dimethyl-N-([$^{18}$F]fluoromethyl)ethanol ammonium; FCHO) have been used to image a wide range of cancers, particularly prostate adenocarcinoma.[86,87] The initial cellular uptake of $^{11}$C-CHO is mediated by choline transporters. There are multiple CHO transporters, including the high-affinity CHO transporter (CHT1, SLC5A7), the intermediate-affinity CHO transporter–like family

(CTLs), organic cation transporters (OCTs), and organic cation/carnitine transporters (OCTNs).[88] Various CHO transporters have been shown to be upregulated in many human cancers, although the specific transporters relevant to imaging gliomas and other brain tumors are not well defined. CHO transporters are active at the BBB,[89] allowing access of $^{11}$C-CHO to nonenhancing regions within gliomas.

The entry of CHO into cells is followed by phosphorylation by choline kinases and subsequent use in phospholipid metabolic pathways, as shown in Fig. 5. Thus, tumor accumulation of $^{11}$C-CHO reflects increased demands for phospholipid synthesis, including membrane synthesis, in tumor cells. Several studies have demonstrated that $^{11}$C-CHO has uptake in gliomas and may assist in tumor grading.[90–92] The boundaries of uptake of $^{11}$C-CHO in high-grade gliomas has been shown to be larger than the area of postgadolinium enhancement on MR imaging, suggesting that this PET tracer is useful for visualizing the nonenhancing regions within glioma.[91]

In a study directly comparing the uptake of $^{11}$C-CHO with $^{11}$C-MET and $^{18}$F-FDG in gliomas, both $^{11}$C-CHO and $^{11}$C-MET demonstrated imaging properties superior to those of $^{18}$F-FDG.[92] In this study of 95 subjects with brain gliomas, $^{11}$C-CHO demonstrated higher but more variable levels of uptake than $^{11}$C-MET in gliomas relative to normal brain, with average tumor to normal brain ratios ranging from approximately 3:1 to 18:1 with $^{11}$C-CHO compared with 2:1 to 5:1 with

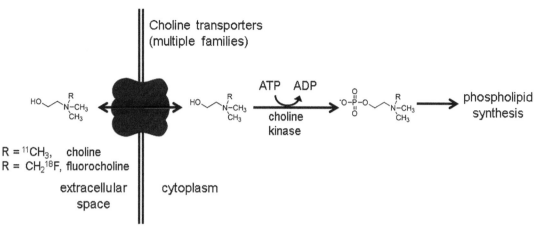

R = $^{11}CH_3$,   choline
R = $CH_2{}^{18}F$, fluorocholine

extracellular          cytoplasm
space

Fig. 5. Cellular uptake and metabolism of $^{11}$C-CHO and $^{18}$F-FCHO. Multiple families of choline transporters mediate the cellular uptake of $^{11}$C-CHO, including the high-affinity CHO transporter (CHT1, SLC5A7), the intermediate-affinity CHO transporter-like family (CTLs), organic cation transporters (OCTs), and organic cation/carnitine transporters (OCTNs), which differ in their transport mechanisms. CHO transport is also active at the BBB. $^{11}$C-CHO is phosphorylated by choline kinases followed by incorporation into phospholipids. $^{18}$F-FCHO is also a substrate for choline transport and choline kinase, and can undergo incorporation into phospholipids, although $^{18}$F-FCHO does not readily cross the BBB.

$^{11}$C-MET. Despite the higher uptake of $^{11}$C-CHO, the investigators concluded that overall, $^{11}$C-MET had more desirable glioma imaging properties, owing to its lower uptake in normal brain structures such as the choroid plexus and pituitary gland.

In a small study with 8 subjects comparing the uptake of $^{11}$C-CHO and $^{11}$C-MET in brain metastases, $^{11}$C-CHO also demonstrated higher lesion to background ratios than $^{11}$C-MET.[93] Another study evaluating the uptake of $^{11}$C-CHO and $^{18}$F-FDG in primary and metastatic brain tumors treated with SRS found that $^{11}$C-CHO was superior to $^{18}$F-FDG in distinguishing radiation necrosis from recurrent tumor.[94] However, the diagnostic significance of this finding and the ability to accurately distinguish recurrent metastases from radiation necrosis remains to be established.

The fluorinated analogue of CHO, $^{18}$F-FCHO, has been developed to take advantage of the longer half-life of fluorine-18.[95] Although FCHO has also shown promise as a tumor imaging agent, it has biochemical and biodistribution properties different from those of $^{11}$C-CHO. The utility of $^{18}$F-FCHO is limited in gliomas because of poor penetration of the BBB, likely due to differences in recognition by transporters at the BBB. There are data suggesting that $^{18}$F-FCHO can distinguish enhancing primary high-grade and metastatic brain tumors from benign enhancing lesions including radiation necrosis.[96] Other studies have shown that nonneoplastic brain lesions, including radiation necrosis, and tumefactive demyelination can have increased uptake of $^{18}$F-FCHO, which

may limit its utility in distinguishing radiation necrosis from recurrent tumor.[97] In a small study of 6 subjects with nonenhancing low-grade gliomas that did not have increased $^{18}$F-FET uptake, $^{18}$F-FCHO also did not demonstrate increased uptake relative to normal brain.[98]

## Acetate

The simple carboxylic acid [$^{11}$C]acetate ($^{11}$C-ACE) has been used extensively for tumor and metabolic imaging in a wide range of applications.[99] $^{11}$C-ACE is a critical metabolic intermediate in cellular metabolism and can serve as a source of energy or as a carbon source for biosynthesis, depending on the cell type. The entry of $^{11}$C-ACE into cells is mediated by monocarboxylate transporters (MCTs) including MCT1 (SLC16A1), MCT2 (SLC16A7), and MCT4 (SLC16A3), which are proton symporters.[100] $^{11}$C-ACE transporters including MCT1 are active at the BBB.[101] In many normal tissues including the myocardium, $^{11}$C-ACE undergoes oxidative metabolism through the tricarboxylic acid (TCA) cycle to form [$^{11}$C]CO$_2$ and water. In many cancer cells, the predominant metabolic pathway for CHO is fatty acid synthesis, with a substantial fraction of the $^{11}$C label being incorporated into cell membranes. There is also evidence in rodent models that nonneoplastic neurons and glial cells as well as gliomas and meningiomas can convert ACE into AAs, including glutamine and glutamate.[100,102] The uptake and potential metabolic fates of $^{11}$C-ACE are shown schematically in **Fig. 6**. There is some evidence

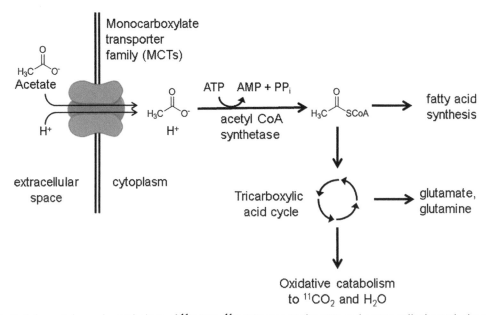

**Fig. 6.** Cellular uptake and metabolism of [11]C-ACE. [11]C-ACE crosses the BBB and enters cells through the mono-carboxylate transporter (MCT) family including MCT1, MCT2, and MCT4. Within cells, [11]C-ACE can undergo oxidative catabolism to produce energy through the tricarboxylic acid (TCA) cycle, or alternatively be incorporated into fatty acids in the cell membranes. In normal brain as well as gliomas and meningiomas, TCA-cycle intermediates derived from [11]C-ACE may be converted into AAs, for example, glutamine and glutamate as well as other metabolic intermediates. AMP, adenosine monophosphate; $PP_i$, inorganic pyrophosphate.

in hepatocellular carcinoma that [11]C-ACE can complement [18]F-FDG through higher uptake than [18]F-FDG in well-differentiated tumors.[103]

The utility of [11]C-ACE PET has been explored through several studies of patients with gliomas and meningiomas. In a study comparing [11]C-ACE with [11]C-MET and [18]F-FDG in patients with brain gliomas, both [11]C-ACE and [11]C-MET had higher tumor to normal brain ratios than [18]F-FDG.[104] In addition, higher SUVs were observed with [11]C-ACE and [18]F-FDG in higher-grade tumors in this study. However, other studies have had conflicting results regarding the utility of [11]C-ACE for grading gliomas.[105,106] In meningiomas, [11]C-ACE was superior to [18]F-FDG for visualization of meningiomas, and demonstrated greater change after SRS than [18]F-FDG.[107] However, the amount of uptake of [11]C-ACE was not useful for distinguishing low-grade from higher-grade meningiomas.

## Somatostatin Receptor PET

Radiolabeled analogues of the naturally occurring somatostatin receptor peptidic ligand, octreotide, have been used extensively for PET and SPECT imaging of neuroendocrine tumors such as carcinoid tumors and pancreatic islet tumors.[108,109] Several analogues have been labeled with gallium-68 for PET, including DOTA-

[Tyr3]-octreotide (DOTATOC) and DOTA-[Tyr3]-octreotate (DOTATATE), which have superior imaging properties than the SPECT agent In-111 pentetreotide, used in routine clinical practice in the United States. The structures of [68]Ga-DOTA-TOC and [68]Ga-DOTATATE are shown in **Fig. 7.** These agents have also been used for therapy by replacing the imaging radionuclide with therapeutic radionuclides such as yttrium-90 and lutetium-177. Like most peptides, these tracers do not cross the intact BBB.

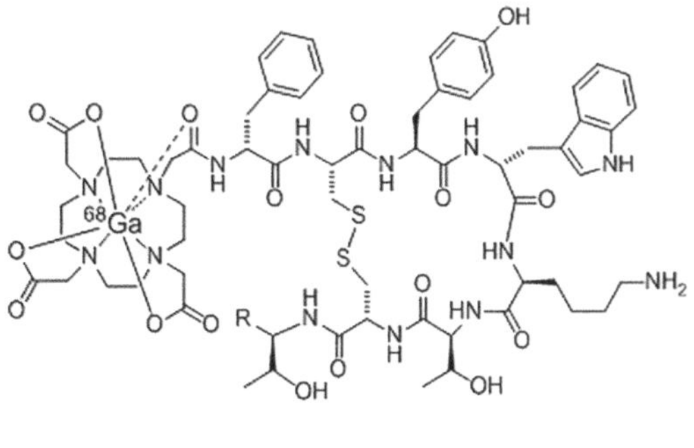

R = CH$_2$OH, DOTATOC

R = CO$_2$H, DOTATATE

**Fig. 7.** Structures of the [68]Ga-labeled somatostatin receptor ligands DOTATOC and DOTATE.

In addition to neuroendocrine tumors, somatostatin receptors are present on approximately 90% of meningiomas,[110] and these tracers are effective imaging agents for meningioma. There is some evidence that [68]Ga-DOTATOC PET can increase the detection of meningiomas by approximately 10% in comparison with MR imaging alone,[111] although the clinical significance of this increased detection rate is unclear. Also, the somatostatin receptor imaging does not appear to distinguish low-grade from high-grade meningiomas. An appealing application of these tracers is for the diagnosis of and therapy for meningiomas, using the same strategy for extra-CNS neuroendocrine tumors when surgical resection and radiotherapy have failed. A recent study using [68]Ga-DOTATATE demonstrated the feasibility of using somatostatin receptor PET for estimating the achievable therapeutic dose in meningiomas with [177]Lu-DOTATATE.[112]

## SUMMARY AND FUTURE DIRECTIONS

A range of PET tracers have been used to image brain tumors in patients, and of these [18]F-FDG, [18]F-FLT, [11]C-MET, and [18]F-FET have the largest amount of supporting data for their efficacy. There are few direct comparisons of the efficacy of non-FDG PET tracers for brain tumor imaging in human studies, but the available data suggest that radiolabeled AAs may be the best suited for estimating gross tumor volumes and margins. There are data supporting the superiority of radiolabeled AAs and [11]C-CHO over [18]F-FDG in distinguishing radiation necrosis from recurrence in patients with primary and metastatic brain tumors, but prospective studies in larger numbers of patients are needed to define the diagnostic accuracy of these techniques. Many of these tracers including [18]F-FDG, [18]F-FLT, and the radiolabeled AAs appear to have some utility in treatment planning and monitoring of response to therapy, but data demonstrating improved patient outcomes through incorporating these tracers into the diagnostic evaluation of neuro-oncology patients is not yet available. Such data are key to gaining regulatory approval and reimbursement for routine clinical use.

Most of the PET tracers that have been successful for brain tumor imaging in humans are small molecules (molecular weight <500 Da) that target different aspects of the altered metabolism present in brain tumors. Other classes of PET tracers including peptides, antibodies, and nanoparticles, as well as tracers targeting single molecular targets such as cell-surface receptors, have received less attention for brain tumor imaging in humans. The preference for small molecules is in part due to BBB permeability considerations, but it is likely that members of these other classes of PET tracers will play important roles in brain tumor imaging in the future. Many of these tracers have the potential to be used for both imaging and therapy, and antibodies and nanoparticles also have the potential for multimodality imaging.

Recent work with [89]Zr-labeled trastuzumab demonstrated good uptake in patients with HER2-positive brain metastases from breast cancer.[113] Preclinical studies suggest that dually labeled derivatives of bevacizumab may be used to image brain tumors with PET and near-infrared fluorescence optical imaging.[114] This type of imaging strategy could be used clinically for noninvasive PET imaging followed by intraoperative guidance using the fluorescent properties of this tracer. Similar monoclonal antibody approaches could be explored for both imaging of and therapy for primary and metastatic brain tumors through the targeting of cell-surface markers. Recent work has shown that peptide-based PET tracers can be used to image gliomas and quantify cell-surface receptors. For example, a [68]Ga-labeled bombesin analogue was used to quantify gastrin-releasing peptide receptor with PET in recurrent gliomas.[115] The main liability of these strategies is the poor BBB penetration of peptides, antibodies, and other large molecules or constructs.

The increasing use of advanced MR imaging and the advent of integrated PET/MR imaging systems will facilitate the optimal use of both modalities for neuro-oncologic imaging.[116–118] This new technology can shorten the overall examination time for patients through simultaneous MR imaging and PET acquisition. The relatively long length of typical MR imaging studies in brain tumors (45–60 minutes) also makes dynamic PET studies using tracers with relatively fast kinetics clinically feasible. Multiparametric analysis of combined PET and MR imaging data may improve diagnostic accuracy in the evaluation of brain tumors before and after therapy. In addition to technological and research advances, fully capitalizing on multimodality imaging will require greater coordination and cross-training between neuroradiologists and nuclear medicine physicians.

In conclusion, a great deal of progress has been made in the development and application of PET tracers for brain tumor imaging. However, significant challenges remain, including optimizing noninvasive tumor grading, guiding the selection of the most appropriate therapeutic regimen, monitoring the response to therapy, and distinguishing viable tumor from treatment effect.

Progress in this field will require further research addressing efficacy and outcomes with existing PET tracers, developing new PET tracers as important novel imaging targets in neuro-oncology are identified, and maximizing the information available through multimodality imaging.

## REFERENCES

1. Keogh BP, Henson JW. Clinical manifestations and diagnostic imaging of brain tumors. Hematol Oncol Clin North Am 2012;26(4):733–55.
2. Upadhyay N, Waldman AD. Conventional MRI evaluation of gliomas. Br J Radiol 2011;84(Spec No 2): S107–11.
3. Wen PY, Kesari S. Malignant gliomas in adults. N Engl J Med 2008;359(5):492–507.
4. Suh JH. Stereotactic radiosurgery for the management of brain metastases. N Engl J Med 2010; 362(12):1119–27.
5. Nayak L, Lee EQ, Wen PY. Epidemiology of brain metastases. Curr Oncol Rep 2012;14(1):48–54.
6. Ferreri AJ, Marturano E. Primary CNS lymphoma. Best Pract Res Clin Haematol 2012;25(1):119–30.
7. Huttner A. Overview of primary brain tumors: pathologic classification, epidemiology, molecular biology, and prognostic markers. Hematol Oncol Clin North Am 2012;26(4):715–32.
8. Patel TR, Knisely JP, Chiang VL. Management of brain metastases: surgery, radiation, or both? Hematol Oncol Clin North Am 2012;26(4):933–47.
9. Ricard D, Idbaih A, Ducray F, et al. Primary brain tumours in adults. Lancet 2012;379(9830):1984–96.
10. Brastianos PK, Batchelor TT. Primary central nervous system lymphoma: overview of current treatment strategies. Hematol Oncol Clin North Am 2012;26(4):897–916.
11. Neuwelt EA, Bauer B, Fahlke C, et al. Engaging neuroscience to advance translational research in brain barrier biology. Nat Rev Neurosci 2011; 12(3):169–82.
12. Thompson EM, Dosa E, Kraemer DF, et al. Correlation of MRI sequences to assess progressive glioblastoma multiforme treated with bevacizumab. J Neurooncol 2011;103(2):353–60.
13. Jain R, Scarpace LM, Ellika S, et al. Imaging response criteria for recurrent gliomas treated with bevacizumab: role of diffusion weighted imaging as an imaging biomarker. J Neurooncol 2010;96(3):423–31.
14. Pauwels EK, Ribeiro MJ, Stoot JH, et al. FDG accumulation and tumor biology. Nucl Med Biol 1998; 25(4):317–22.
15. Simpson IA, Appel NM, Hokari M, et al. Blood-brain barrier glucose transporter: effects of hypo- and hyperglycemia revisited. J Neurochem 1999; 72(1):238–47.

16. Chen W. Clinical applications of PET in brain tumors. J Nucl Med 2007;48(9):1468–81.
17. Padma MV, Said S, Jacobs M, et al. Prediction of pathology and survival by FDG PET in gliomas. J Neurooncol 2003;64(3):227–37.
18. Dequesada IM, Quisling RG, Yachnis A, et al. Can standard magnetic resonance imaging reliably distinguish recurrent tumor from radiation necrosis after radiosurgery for brain metastases? A radiographic-pathological study. Neurosurgery 2008;63(5):898–903 [discussion: 904].
19. Shah R, Vattoth S, Jacob R, et al. Radiation necrosis in the brain: imaging features and differentiation from tumor recurrence. Radiographics 2012;32(5):1343–59.
20. Kahn D, Follett KA, Bushnell DL, et al. Diagnosis of recurrent brain tumor: value of [201]Tl SPECT vs [18]F-fluorodeoxyglucose PET. AJR Am J Roentgenol 1994;163(6):1459–65.
21. Siepmann DB, Siegel A, Lewis PJ. Tl-201 SPECT and F-18 FDG PET for assessment of glioma recurrence versus radiation necrosis. Clin Nucl Med 2005;30(3):199–200.
22. Asao C, Korogi Y, Kitajima M, et al. Diffusion-weighted imaging of radiation-induced brain injury for differentiation from tumor recurrence. AJNR Am J Neuroradiol 2005;26(6):1455–60.
23. Larsen VA, Simonsen HJ, Law I, et al. Evaluation of dynamic contrast-enhanced T1-weighted perfusion MRI in the differentiation of tumor recurrence from radiation necrosis. Neuroradiology 2012. http://dx.doi.org/10.1007/s00234-012-1127-4. [Epub ahead of print].
24. Horky LL, Hsiao EM, Weiss SE, et al. Dual phase FDG-PET imaging of brain metastases provides superior assessment of recurrence versus post-treatment necrosis. J Neurooncol 2011;103(1): 137–46.
25. O'Doherty MJ, Barrington SF, Campbell M, et al. PET scanning and the human immunodeficiency virus-positive patient. J Nucl Med 1997;38(10):1575–83.
26. Hustinx R, Smith RJ, Benard F, et al. Can the standardized uptake value characterize primary brain tumors on FDG-PET? Eur J Nucl Med 1999; 26(11):1501–9.
27. Kostakoglu L. Novel PET radiotracers for potential use in management of lymphoma. PET Clin 2012; 7:83–117.
28. Plotnik DA, Emerick LE, Krohn KA, et al. Different modes of transport for [3]H-thymidine, [3]H-FLT, and [3]H-FMAU in proliferating and nonproliferating human tumor cells. J Nucl Med 2010;51(9):1464–71.
29. Barthel H, Perumal M, Latigo J, et al. The uptake of 3'-deoxy-3'-[[18]F]fluorothymidine into L5178Y tumours in vivo is dependent on thymidine kinase 1 protein levels. Eur J Nucl Med Mol Imaging 2005;32(3):257–63.

30. Shields AF, Grierson JR, Dohmen BM, et al. Imaging proliferation in vivo with [F-18]FLT and positron emission tomography. Nat Med 1998; 4(11):1334–6.

31. Buchmann I, Neumaier B, Schreckenberger M, et al. [18F]3′-deoxy-3′-fluorothymidine-PET in NHL patients: whole-body biodistribution and imaging of lymphoma manifestations–a pilot study. Cancer Biother Radiopharm 2004;19(4):436–42.

32. Idema AJ, Hoffmann AL, Boogaarts HD, et al. 3′-Deoxy-3′-18F-fluorothymidine PET-derived proliferative volume predicts overall survival in high-grade glioma patients. J Nucl Med 2012;53(12):1904–10.

33. Chen W, Cloughesy T, Kamdar N, et al. Imaging proliferation in brain tumors with 18F-FLT PET: comparison with 18F-FDG. J Nucl Med 2005; 46(6):945–52.

34. Miyake K, Shinomiya A, Okada M, et al. Usefulness of FDG, MET and FLT-PET studies for the management of human gliomas. J Biomed Biotechnol 2012; 2012:205818.

35. Price SJ, Fryer TD, Cleij MC, et al. Imaging regional variation of cellular proliferation in gliomas using 3′-deoxy-3′-[18F]fluorothymidine positron-emission tomography: an image-guided biopsy study. Clin Radiol 2009;64(1):52–63.

36. Chen W, Delaloye S, Silverman DH, et al. Predicting treatment response of malignant gliomas to bevacizumab and irinotecan by imaging proliferation with [18F] fluorothymidine positron emission tomography: a pilot study. J Clin Oncol 2007;25(30): 4714–21.

37. Harris RJ, Cloughesy TF, Pope WB, et al. 18F-FDOPA and 18F-FLT positron emission tomography parametric response maps predict response in recurrent malignant gliomas treated with bevacizumab. Neuro Oncol 2012;14(8):1079–89.

38. Tripathi M, Sharma R, D'Souza M, et al. Comparative evaluation of F-18 FDOPA, F-18 FDG, and F-18 FLT-PET/CT for metabolic imaging of low grade gliomas. Clin Nucl Med 2009;34(12):878–83.

39. Choi SJ, Kim JS, Kim JH, et al. [18F]3′-deoxy-3′-fluorothymidine PET for the diagnosis and grading of brain tumors. Eur J Nucl Med Mol Imaging 2005; 32(6):653–9.

40. Jager PL, Vaalburg W, Pruim J, et al. Radiolabeled amino acids: basic aspects and clinical applications in oncology. J Nucl Med 2001;42(3):432–45.

41. McConathy J, Yu WP, Jarkas N, et al. Radiohalogenated nonnatural amino acids as PET and SPECT tumor imaging agents. Med Res Rev 2012;32(4):868–905.

42. Verrey F, Closs EI, Wagner CA, et al. CATs and HATs: the SLC7 family of amino acid transporters. Pflugers Arch 2004;447(5):532–42.

43. Mackenzie B, Erickson JD. Sodium-coupled neutral amino acid (System N/A) transporters of the SLC38 gene family. Pflugers Arch 2004; 447(5):784–95.

44. Langen KJ, Broer S. Molecular transport mechanisms of radiolabeled amino acids for PET and SPECT. J Nucl Med 2004;45(9):1435–6.

45. Kanai Y, Hediger MA. The glutamate/neutral amino acid transporter family SLC1: molecular, physiological and pharmacological aspects. Pflugers Arch 2004;447(5):469–79.

46. Verrey F. System L: heteromeric exchangers of large, neutral amino acids involved in directional transport. Pflugers Arch 2003;445(5):529–33.

47. Palacin M, Estevez R, Bertran J, et al. Molecular biology of mammalian plasma membrane amino acid transporters. Physiol Rev 1998; 78(4):969–1054.

48. Matsuo H, Tsukada S, Nakata T, et al. Expression of a system L neutral amino acid transporter at the blood-brain barrier. Neuroreport 2000;11(16): 3507–11.

49. Haining Z, Kawai N, Miyake K, et al. Relation of LAT1/4F2hc expression with pathological grade, proliferation and angiogenesis in human gliomas. BMC Clin Pathol 2012;12:4.

50. Nawashiro H, Otani N, Shinomiya N, et al. L-type amino acid transporter 1 as a potential molecular target in human astrocytic tumors. Int J Cancer 2006;119(3):484–92.

51. Fuchs BC, Bode BP. Amino acid transporters ASCT2 and LAT1 in cancer: partners in crime? Semin Cancer Biol 2005;15(4):254–66.

52. Singhal T, Narayanan TK, Jain V, et al. [11C]-L-methionine positron emission tomography in the clinical management of cerebral gliomas. Mol Imaging Biol 2008;10(1):1–18.

53. Langen KJ, Hamacher K, Weckesser M, et al. O-(2-[18F]fluoroethyl)-L-tyrosine: uptake mechanisms and clinical applications. Nucl Med Biol 2006; 33(3):287–94.

54. Chen W, Silverman DH, Delaloye S, et al. 18F-FDOPA PET imaging of brain tumors: comparison study with 18F-FDG PET and evaluation of diagnostic accuracy. J Nucl Med 2006;47(6):904–11.

55. Grosu AL, Astner ST, Riedel E, et al. An interindividual comparison of (2-[18F]fluoroethyl)-L-tyrosine (FET)- and L-[methyl-11C]methionine (MET)-PET in patients with brain gliomas and metastases. Int J Radiat Oncol Biol Phys 2011;81(4):1049–58.

56. Miwa K, Shinoda J, Yano H, et al. Discrepancy between lesion distributions on methionine PET and MR images in patients with glioblastoma multiforme: insight from a PET and MR fusion image study. J Neurol Neurosurg Psychiatry 2004; 75(10):1457–62.

57. Kracht LW, Miletic H, Busch S, et al. Delineation of brain tumor extent with [11C]L-methionine positron emission tomography: local comparison with

stereotactic histopathology. Clin Cancer Res 2004;10(21):7163–70.

58. Plotkin M, Blechschmidt C, Auf G, et al. Comparison of F-18 FET-PET with F-18 FDG-PET for biopsy planning of non-contrast-enhancing gliomas. Eur Radiol 2010;20(10):2496–502.

59. Pauleit D, Floeth F, Hamacher K, et al. O-(2-[18F]fluoroethyl)-L-tyrosine PET combined with MRI improves the diagnostic assessment of cerebral gliomas. Brain 2005;128(Pt 3):678–87.

60. Calcagni ML, Galli G, Giordano A, et al. Dynamic O-(2-[18F]fluoroethyl)-L-tyrosine (F-18 FET) PET for glioma grading: assessment of individual probability of malignancy. Clin Nucl Med 2011;36(10): 841–7.

61. Popperl G, Kreth FW, Mehrkens JH, et al. FET PET for the evaluation of untreated gliomas: correlation of FET uptake and uptake kinetics with tumour grading. Eur J Nucl Med Mol Imaging 2007; 34(12):1933–42.

62. Popperl G, Kreth FW, Herms J, et al. Analysis of 18F-FET PET for grading of recurrent gliomas: is evaluation of uptake kinetics superior to standard methods? J Nucl Med 2006;47(3):393–403.

63. Wyss M, Hofer S, Bruehlmeier M, et al. Early metabolic responses in temozolomide treated lowgrade glioma patients. J Neurooncol 2009;95(1): 87–93.

64. Ribom D, Schoenmaekers M, Engler H, et al. Evaluation of 11C-methionine PET as a surrogate endpoint after treatment of grade 2 gliomas. J Neurooncol 2005;71(3):325–32.

65. Kim YH, Oh SW, Lim YJ, et al. Differentiating radiation necrosis from tumor recurrence in high-grade gliomas: assessing the efficacy of 18F-FDG PET, 11C-methionine PET and perfusion MRI. Clin Neurol Neurosurg 2010;112(9):758–65.

66. Nakajima T, Kumabe T, Kanamori M, et al. Differential diagnosis between radiation necrosis and glioma progression using sequential proton magnetic resonance spectroscopy and methionine positron emission tomography. Neurol Med Chir (Tokyo) 2009;49(9):394–401.

67. Terakawa Y, Tsuyuguchi N, Iwai Y, et al. Diagnostic accuracy of 11C-methionine PET for differentiation of recurrent brain tumors from radiation necrosis after radiotherapy. J Nucl Med 2008;49(5):694–9.

68. Langen KJ, Jarosch M, Hamacher K, et al. Imaging of gliomas with Cis-4-[18F]fluoro-L-proline. Nucl Med Biol 2004;31(1):67–75.

69. Betz AL, Goldstein GW. Polarity of the blood-brain barrier: neutral amino acid transport into isolated brain capillaries. Science 1978;202(4364):225–7.

70. Yu W, McConathy J, Williams L, et al. Synthesis, radiolabeling, and biological evaluation of (R)- and (S)-2-amino-3-[(18)F]fluoro-2-methylpropanoic acid (FAMP) and (R)- and (S)-3-[(18)F]fluoro-2-methyl-2-

N-(methylamino)propanoic acid (MMeFAMP) as potential PET radioligands for imaging brain tumors. J Med Chem 2010;53(2):876–86.

71. Yu W, McConathy J, Olson J, et al. Facile stereospecific synthesis and biological evaluation of (S)- and (R)-2-Amino-2-methyl-4-[123I]iodo-3-(E)-butenoic acid for brain tumor imaging with single photon emission computerized tomography. J Med Chem 2007;50(26):6718–21.

72. McConathy J, Martarello L, Malveaux EJ, et al. Radiolabeled amino acids for tumor imaging with PET: radiosynthesis and biological evaluation of 2-amino-3-[18F]fluoro-2-methylpropanoic acid and 3-[18F]fluoro-2-methyl-2-(methylamino)propanoic acid. J Med Chem 2002;45(11):2240–9.

73. Qu W, Oya S, Lieberman BP, et al. Preparation and characterization of L-[5-11C]-glutamine for metabolic imaging of tumors. J Nucl Med 2012;53(1): 98–105.

74. Lieberman BP, Ploessl K, Wang L, et al. PET imaging of glutaminolysis in tumors by 18F-(2S,4R)-4-fluoroglutamine. J Nucl Med 2011; 52(12):1947–55.

75. Krasikova RN, Kuznetsova OF, Fedorova OS, et al. 4-[18F]fluoroglutamic acid (BAY 85-8050), a new amino acid radiotracer for PET imaging of tumors: synthesis and in vitro characterization. J Med Chem 2011;54(1):406–10.

76. Savaskan NE, Eyupoglu IY. xCT modulation in gliomas: relevance to energy metabolism and tumor microenvironment normalization. Ann Anat 2010;192(5):309–13.

77. McConathy J, Zhou D, Shockley SE, et al. Click synthesis and biologic evaluation of (R)- and (S)-2-Amino-3-[1-(2-[18F]fluoroethyl)-1H-[1,2,3]Triazol-4-yl]propanoic acid for brain tumor imaging with positron emission tomography. Mol Imaging 2010; 9(6):329–42.

78. Padhani A. PET imaging of tumour hypoxia. Cancer Imaging 2006;6:S117–21.

79. Kurihara H, Honda N, Kono Y, et al. Radiolabelled agents for PET imaging of tumor hypoxia. Curr Med Chem 2012;19(20):3282–9.

80. Hirata K, Terasaka S, Shiga T, et al. 18F-Fluoromisonidazole positron emission tomography may differentiate glioblastoma multiforme from less malignant gliomas. Eur J Nucl Med Mol Imaging 2012;39(5):760–70.

81. Swanson KR, Chakraborty G, Wang CH, et al. Complementary but distinct roles for MRI and 18F-fluoromisonidazole PET in the assessment of human glioblastomas. J Nucl Med 2009;50(1):36–44.

82. Mendichovszky I, Jackson A. Imaging hypoxia in gliomas. Br J Radiol 2011;84(Spec No 2):S145–58.

83. Szeto MD, Chakraborty G, Hadley J, et al. Quantitative metrics of net proliferation and invasion link biological aggressiveness assessed by MRI with

hypoxia assessed by FMISO-PET in newly diagnosed glioblastomas. Cancer Res 2009;69(10): 4502–9.

84. Spence AM, Muzi M, Swanson KR, et al. Regional hypoxia in glioblastoma multiforme quantified with [18F]fluoromisonidazole positron emission tomography before radiotherapy: correlation with time to progression and survival. Clin Cancer Res 2008; 14(9):2623–30.

85. Tateishi K, Tateishi U, Sato M, et al. Application of 62Cu-Diacetyl-Bis (N4-Methylthiosemicarbazone) PET imaging to predict highly malignant tumor grades and hypoxia-inducible factor-1alpha expression in patients with glioma. AJNR Am J Neuroradiol 2013;34(1):92–9.

86. Treglia G, Giovannini E, Di Franco D, et al. The role of positron emission tomography using carbon-11 and fluorine-18 choline in tumors other than prostate cancer: a systematic review. Ann Nucl Med 2012;26(6):451–61.

87. Mertens K, Slaets D, Lambert B, et al. PET with (18) F-labelled choline-based tracers for tumour imaging: a review of the literature. Eur J Nucl Med Mol Imaging 2010;37(11):2188–93.

88. Glunde K, Bhujwalla ZM, Ronen SM. Choline metabolism in malignant transformation. Nat Rev Cancer 2011;11(12):835–48.

89. Allen DD, Smith QR. Characterization of the blood-brain barrier choline transporter using the in situ rat brain perfusion technique. J Neurochem 2001; 76(4):1032–41.

90. Tian M, Zhang H, Oriuchi N, et al. Comparison of 11C-choline PET and FDG PET for the differential diagnosis of malignant tumors. Eur J Nucl Med Mol Imaging 2004;31(8):1064–72.

91. Ohtani T, Kurihara H, Ishiuchi S, et al. Brain tumour imaging with carbon-11 choline: comparison with FDG PET and gadolinium-enhanced MR imaging. Eur J Nucl Med 2001;28(11):1664–70.

92. Kato T, Shinoda J, Nakayama N, et al. Metabolic assessment of gliomas using 11C-methionine, [18F] fluorodeoxyglucose, and 11C-choline positron-emission tomography. AJNR Am J Neuroradiol 2008;29(6):1176–82.

93. Rottenburger C, Hentschel M, Kelly T, et al. Comparison of C-11 methionine and C-11 choline for PET imaging of brain metastases: a prospective pilot study. Clin Nucl Med 2011; 36(8):639–42.

94. Tan H, Chen L, Guan Y, et al. Comparison of MRI, F-18 FDG, and 11C-choline PET/CT for their potentials in differentiating brain tumor recurrence from brain tumor necrosis following radiotherapy. Clin Nucl Med 2011;36(11):978–81.

95. Kwee SA, DeGrado TR, Talbot JN, et al. Cancer imaging with fluorine-18-labeled choline derivatives. Semin Nucl Med 2007;37(6):420–8.

96. Kwee SA, Ko JP, Jiang CS, et al. Solitary brain lesions enhancing at MR imaging: evaluation with fluorine 18 fluorocholine PET. Radiology 2007; 244(2):557–65.

97. Mertens K, Bolcaen J, Ham H, et al. The optimal timing for imaging brain tumours and other brain lesions with 18F-labelled fluoromethylcholine: a dynamic positron emission tomography study. Nucl Med Commun 2012;33(9):954–9.

98. Roelcke U, Bruehlmeier M, Hefti M, et al. F-18 choline PET does not detect increased metabolism in F-18 fluoroethyltyrosine-negative low-grade gliomas. Clin Nucl Med 2012;37(1):e1–3.

99. Grassi I, Nanni C, Allegri V, et al. The clinical use of PET with (11)C-acetate. Am J Nucl Med Mol Imaging 2012;2(1):33–47.

100. Rae C, Fekete AD, Kashem MA, et al. Metabolism, compartmentation, transport and production of acetate in the cortical brain tissue slice. Neurochem Res 2012;37(11):2541–53.

101. Halestrap AP, Wilson MC. The monocarboxylate transporter family–role and regulation. IUBMB Life 2012;64(2):109–19.

102. Dienel GA, Popp D, Drew PD, et al. Preferential labeling of glial and meningeal brain tumors with [2-(14)C]acetate. J Nucl Med 2001;42(8):1243–50.

103. Park JW, Kim JH, Kim SK, et al. A prospective evaluation of 18F-FDG and 11C-acetate PET/CT for detection of primary and metastatic hepatocellular carcinoma. J Nucl Med 2008;49(12):1912–21.

104. Yamamoto Y, Nishiyama Y, Kimura N, et al. 11C-acetate PET in the evaluation of brain glioma: comparison with 11C-methionine and 18F-FDG-PET. Mol Imaging Biol 2008;10(5):281–7.

105. Tsuchida T, Takeuchi H, Okazawa H, et al. Grading of brain glioma with 1-11C-acetate PET: comparison with 18F-FDG PET. Nucl Med Biol 2008;35(2):171–6.

106. Liu RS, Chang CP, Chu LS, et al. PET imaging of brain astrocytoma with 1-11C-acetate. Eur J Nucl Med Mol Imaging 2006;33(4):420–7.

107. Liu RS, Chang CP, Guo WY, et al. 1-11C-acetate versus 18F-FDG PET in detection of meningioma and monitoring the effect of gamma-knife radiosurgery. J Nucl Med 2010;51(6):883–91.

108. Treglia G, Castaldi P, Rindi G, et al. Diagnostic performance of Gallium-68 somatostatin receptor PET and PET/CT in patients with thoracic and gastroenteropancreatic neuroendocrine tumours: a meta-analysis. Endocrine 2012;42(1):80–7.

109. Baum RP, Kulkarni HR, Carreras C. Peptides and receptors in image-guided therapy: theranostics for neuroendocrine neoplasms. Semin Nucl Med 2012;42(3):190–207.

110. Arena S, Barbieri F, Thellung S, et al. Expression of somatostatin receptor mRNA in human meningiomas and their implication in in vitro antiproliferative activity. J Neurooncol 2004;66(1–2):155–66.

111. Afshar-Oromieh A, Giesel FL, Linhart HG, et al. Detection of cranial meningiomas: comparison of $^{68}$Ga-DOTATOC PET/CT and contrast-enhanced MRI. Eur J Nucl Med Mol Imaging 2012;39(9): 1409–15.

112. Hanscheid H, Sweeney RA, Flentje M, et al. PET SUV correlates with radionuclide uptake in peptide receptor therapy in meningioma. Eur J Nucl Med Mol Imaging 2012;39(8):1284–8.

113. Dijkers EC, Oude Munnink TH, Kosterink JG, et al. Biodistribution of $^{89}$Zr-trastuzumab and PET imaging of HER2-positive lesions in patients with metastatic breast cancer. Clin Pharmacol Ther 2010;87(5):586–92.

114. Zhang Y, Hong H, Engle JW, et al. Positron emission tomography and near-infrared fluorescence imaging of vascular endothelial growth factor with dual-labeled bevacizumab. Am J Nucl Med Mol Imaging 2012;2(1):1–13.

115. Strauss LG, Koczan D, Seiz M, et al. Correlation of the Ga-68-bombesin analog Ga-68-BZH3 with receptors expression in gliomas as measured by quantitative dynamic positron emission tomography (dPET) and gene arrays. Mol Imaging Biol 2012;14(3):376–83.

116. Shah NJ, Oros-Peusquens AM, Arrubla J, et al. Advances in multimodal neuroimaging: hybrid MR-PET and MR-PET-EEG at 3T and 9.4T. J Magn Reson 2012. http://dx.doi.org/10.1016/j.jmr.2012. 11.027. [Epub ahead of print].

117. Neuner I, Kaffanke JB, Langen KJ, et al. Multimodal imaging utilising integrated MR-PET for human brain tumour assessment. Eur Radiol 2012;22(12):2568–80.

118. Bisdas S, Ritz R, Bender B, et al. Metabolic mapping of gliomas using hybrid MR-PET imaging: feasibility of the method and spatial distribution of metabolic changes. Invest Radiol 2013. http://dx.doi.org/10. 1097/RLI.0b013e31827188d6. [Epub ahead of print].

# FET PET in Neuro-oncology and in Evaluation of Treatment Response

Vincent Dunet, BSc, MD[a,b], John O. Prior, PhD, MD[a,*]

## KEYWORDS

• PET • F-18-fluoroethyltyrosine • FET • Amino acid PET • Brain tumor • Glioma

## KEY POINTS

- Molecular imaging with [18]F-fluoroethyltyrosine (FET) PET helps in vivo tumor delineation and grade estimation. It may be used for treatment planning and early detection of residual tumor.
- FET PET assists in selecting the biopsy site in non–contrast-enhancing tumors, which are in half of patients of high grade III–IV, thus helping to decrease the probability of undertreatment.
- FET PET may aid in assessing treatment response and solving the progression versus pseudoprogression (radiation necrosis) dilemma and is of prognostic value.
- FET PET has the potential to change clinical management, most often from "watchful waiting" to "treat now"; this needs to be evaluated in terms of patient survival.
- Pitfalls (positive/negative FET lesions) are to be known from nuclear medicine physicians to obtain a correct diagnosis; combining PET with a recent MR image and performing integrated multimodality interpretation with a neuroradiologist can be of interest.
- Evidences for cost efficiency of adding FET PET to MR imaging are in development in (1) guiding surgical resection of high-grade glioma and (2) guiding target selection for biopsy to diagnose glioma.

## INTRODUCTION

Primary brain tumors represent 1% to 2% of all adult cancers in the United States, with almost 230,000 central nervous system tumors diagnosed between 2004 and 2007.[1] Among primary brain tumors, gliomas constitute the most frequent pathologic finding, being characterized by distinct histologic patterns and grades that are predictive of tumor invasiveness and patient survival. Morphologic assessment by magnetic resonance (MR) imaging is often the first step toward diagnosis of primary brain tumor, allowing precise assessment of tumor size, limits, mass effect, and presence or absence of contrast enhancement.

However, it lacks specificity and does not allow the determination of tumor metabolism and activity. MR spectroscopy constitutes a step further and allows assessing the presence of neuronal and membrane metabolites but has poor spatial resolution and is often limited by the proximity of bone or artifacts produced by cerebrospinal liquid.

Molecular imaging with PET provides information on tumor metabolism and allows the identification of zones of increased growth activity. Because [18]F-fluorodeoxyglucose (FDG) uptake is high in the normal brain and unspecifically associated with inflammation, PET with [18]F-FDG is an

Disclosure: The authors have no relationship to disclose. [18]F-fluoroethyltyrosine (FET) has not received FDA approval.
a Department of Nuclear Medicine, Lausanne University Hospital, Rue du Bugnon 46, Lausanne 1011, Switzerland; b Department of Radiology, Lausanne University Hospital, Rue du Bugnon 46, Lausanne 1011, Switzerland
* Corresponding author.
E-mail address: John.Prior@chuv.ch

PET Clin 8 (2013) 147–162
http://dx.doi.org/10.1016/j.cpet.2012.09.005
1556-8598/13/$ – see front matter © 2013 Elsevier Inc. All rights reserved.

pet.theclinics.com

inadequate and unreliable tool to prove the tumoral nature of a lesion in the brain, in particular in lower-grade tumors. In contrast, amino acid tracers provide images with a high contrast-to-noise ratio. Developed more than a decade ago, the PET radiotracer [18]F-fluoroethyltyrosine (FET) demonstrates good sensitivity and specificity to diagnose primary brain tumor, probe tumoral biologic growth, assess tumor response to therapy, and detect tumor recurrence. This review describes the role of FET PET in the management of patients with suspected or proved primary brain tumors (**Box 1**) and highlights future perspectives.

## NORMAL ANATOMY/IMAGING TECHNIQUE
### Tracer Biology, Uptake Mechanism, and Physiologic Pattern

FET is an artificial amino acid (chemical structure, O-(2-[F-18]fluoroethyl)-L-tyrosine), first synthesized by Wester and colleagues[2] based on the [18]F-fluoroalkylation of the disodium salt of L-tyrosine. Different methods providing high radiochemical purity and high in vitro stability have been described since. Labeling with [18]F allows its use in institutions with no access to a cyclotron, in contrast to [11]C-methionine, one of the first radiolabeled amino acids. FET PET imaging is routinely used at many institutions throughout Europe, and no adverse side effects have been reported. It is not approved by the United States Food and Drug Administration and therefore not used in North America; the natural amino acid 3,4-dihydroxy-[18F]fluorophenylalanine has been used for tumor grading at diagnosis, but this compound has an inherently high uptake in the striatum.[3]

In mice, FET rapidly (<10 minutes) accumulates in the pancreas and moderately in the liver, spleen, lung, muscles, colon, and kidney, followed by continuous renal clearance without renal reuptake.[4] FET is also taken up early by normal brain

tissue, with retention for approximately 1 hour postinjection and then progressive clearance comparable to other organs. In humans, FET kinetics is similar except that pancreas and muscles have a much lower or higher uptake, respectively.[5] FET is continuously eliminated in the urine, reaching a urinary excretion rate of 5% per hour. The percentage of urinary intact FET has been reported as $72 \pm 5\%$ at 1 hour, in accordance with good in vivo stability. Low uptake is seen in the bone, bone marrow, biliary tract, lung parenchyma, myocardium, and thyroid (**Fig. 1**). In the brain, FET uptake increases in normal gray and white matter to reach a plateau 20 minutes postinjection and the value remains stable until 120 minutes postinjection (**Fig. 2**).[5,6]

In brain tumors, FET kinetics depends on histology and grade. FET is taken up into upregulated neoplastic cells but is not incorporated into proteins, in contrast to natural amino acids such as [11]C-methionine, which has a 15% incorporation rate.[2,4] The FET tracer uptake mechanism is complex and not fully understood. Studies demonstrated an FET uptake via a $Na^+$-independent system L and $Na^+$-dependent system $B^{0,+}$ and $B^0$. Langen and colleagues[7] demonstrated a 70% system L and a 30% $Na^+$-dependent system FET uptake in F98 rat glioma cells. System L presents different transporter subtypes (LAT1, LAT2, and LAT3), LAT1 being the first described in C6 rat glioma cells. Babu and colleagues[8] demonstrated that LAT3 was only a poor nonspecific transporter of L-tyrosine. Recent studies highlight that inflammatory tissues do not explain LAT2, suggesting a potential explanation for the lower uptake of FET by inflammatory cells than [11]C-methionine or [18]F-FDG. Regarding the uptake correlation between [11]C-methionine and FET and between [11]C-methionine uptake and LAT1 expression in human glioma,[9] there are growing evidences for an LAT1 involvement in FET uptake. The

---

**Box 1**
**FET PET indications**

- Tumor delineation and characterization (grading)
- Selection of the best site for biopsy in heterogeneous tumors without noncontrast enhancement on MR
- Therapy planning (surgery or radiation therapy)
- Early detection of residual tumor after resection
- Early assessment of tumor response to radiation therapy or chemotherapy
- Detection of tumor grade transformation
- Differentiation of progression versus pseudoprogression (tumor relapse vs radiation necrosis)
- Prognosis

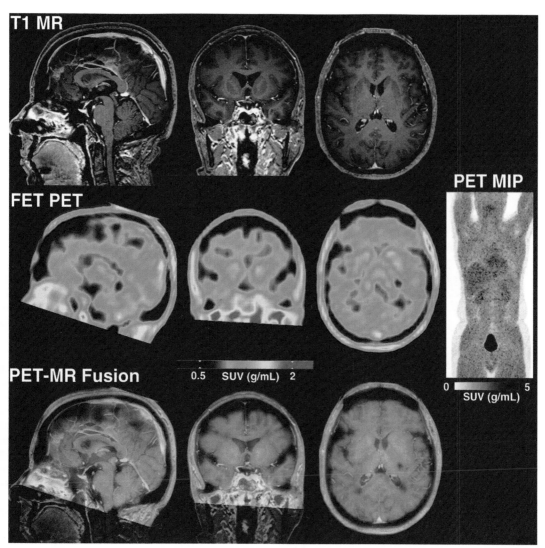

**Fig. 1.** Normal FET PET (50- to 60-minute image frame; $SUV_{max}$ = 1.2 g/mL in striatum, 1.1 g/mL in gray matter, 0.9 g/mL in white matter, 0.8 g/mL in cerebrospinal fluid, and 1.5 g/mL in sagittal venous sinus). On the trunk acquisition (PET maximal intensity projection [MIP] image), FET is mainly concentrated in the kidneys, muscles, liver, spleen, pancreas, and mediastinum, with a medium-range uptake ($SUV_{max}$ = 2–3 g/mL), and it is excreted through the bladder. No significant uptake is seen in the lungs or bone ($SUV_{max}$ = 0.5–0.8 g/mL).

intracellular transport mechanism of FET seems thus to involve multiple pathways, including the specific LAT1 subtype system and the ubiquitous $Na^+$-dependent system $B^{0,+}$ and $B^0$.

## Imaging Protocol

To provide good image quality and ensure reproducibility of the examination, the patient should be carefully prepared (**Box 2**). European guidelines recommend a fasting state for at least 4 hours before FET PET[10] to avoid saturation with unlabeled L-amino acid modifying FET transport into tumor cells.[11]

After injection, PET images are dynamically acquired for about 40 to 60 minutes (8–12 frames of 5 minutes or 4–6 frames of 10 minutes). For analysis, reorientation following the anterior commissure- posterior commissure (AC-PC) line and orthogonal planes reformates are used to ensure precise lesion localization, or fusion images are frequently generated with recent T1-weighted and T2-weighted MR images.

## Image Analysis

FET PET image analysis provides both qualitative and quantitative information. The use of last acquired averaged frames (40–50 or 50–60

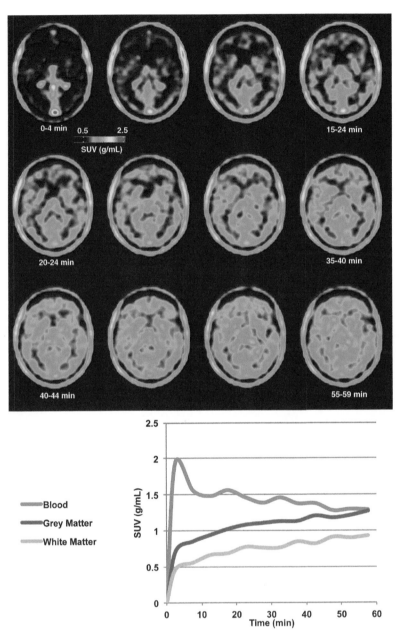

**Fig. 2.** Normal FET dynamic acquisition from 0 to 60 minutes in 5-minute frames with corresponding time–activity curves (SUV$_{max}$) in different brain regions.

minutes) allows the reduction of brain–blood noise and improves the signal-to-noise ratio. Lesion maximum and mean standard uptake value (SUV) can thus be determined on average frames images. Moreover, by measuring the contralateral normal brain uptake, maximum and mean tumor-to-background ratios (TBR$_{max}$, TBR$_{mean}$) may be derived. For computing SUV and TBR, several techniques have been proposed in the literature, such as a region of interest (ROI) manually drawn around the tumor based on increased FET uptake[12–14] or automated ROI drawing based on area with increased FET uptake more than 3 standard deviations of the mean SUV of the control region.[15] By reporting ROI on each slice, a volume of interest (VOI) around the tumor is defined, which is reported on each frame of the dynamic acquisition to determine time–activity curves, allowing for differentiation between low- and high-grade gliomas (**Box 3**).

---

**Box 2**
**Image acquisition protocols for FET PET**

*Recommended FET PET patient preparation and image acquisition*

- Patient preparation: fasting for more than 4 hours + drinking of 1 L water before PET; no glucose restriction needed

- PET: Patient is installed comfortably with appropriate headrest and should void right before PET and directly after image acquisition

- Injection: 200 to 250 MBq in adults; in children, refer to the European Association of Nuclear Medicine dosage card (http://www.eanm.org/docs/dosagecard.pdf, class B radiotracer). Effective dose = 16.5 μSv/MBq for a 70-kg adult (3.3 mSv for 200 MBq); highest absorbed doses in bladder (60 μGy/MBq)[5]

- Women in child-bearing age: perform a pregnancy test; breast-feeding mothers need to stop for more than 12 hours and draw their milk (which should be thrown- away)

- Dynamic image acquisition: 3-dimensional mode starting with an injection for 8 to 10 frames × 5 minutes; check for patient movement; 128 × 128 pixel images corrected for attenuation, reconstructed with ordered subset expectation maximization or filtered back projection; check for patient movement

- Quantitative evaluation: TBR is computed from the 20- to 40-minute image by dividing the $SUV_{max}$ of the lesion by the $SUV_{mean}$ in a background normal reference region (contralateral to the lesion or away from it if located on the midline): $TBR = SUV_{max}/SUV_{mean}$; $TBR \geq 1.6$ is considered to characterize neoplastic region by FET

- Report the (1) time frame and the method used to compute SUV; (2) description of the localization and heterogeneity of FET uptake; (3) possible sources of artifacts (patient movement and small lesions) or known FET-negative lesions (eg, 20%–30% of low-grade glioma); (4) if possible, perform PET–MR fusion and common readout with neuroradiologists

*Abbreviations:* SUV, standard uptake value; TBR, tumor-to-background ratio.

## IMAGES FINDINGS/PATHOLOGY
### Diagnosis of Primary Brain Tumor

Numerous but usually small studies assessed FET PET value in the diagnosis of primary brain tumors.

FET PET was shown to be more accurate than [123]I-iodo-α-methyltyrosine single photon emission computed tomography,[13] [18]F-FDG,[16,17] [18]F-fluorothymidine,[18] and [18]F-fluorocholine[19] PET to detect brain tumor.

---

**Box 3**
**Diagnostic criteria for grading gliomas on FET PET**

| Diagnostic Criteria for Glioma | |
|---|---|
| **Low grade (WHO I–II)** | **High grade (WHO III–IV)** |
| FET uptake higher than in normal brain: $TBR_{mean} \geq 1.7$ or $TBR_{max} \geq 2.1$ | |
| Observe **FET uptake on time–activity curve** | |
| Late (>15 minutes) maximal uptake followed by cumulative curve | Early (≤15 minutes) maximal uptake followed by decreasing curve |
| Compute the **early-to-middle SUV ratio** in tumor (derived from[22]): e-m ratio = $SUV_{5-10\ min}/SUV_{30-35\ min}$ | |
| e-m ratio <0.90 | e-m ratio ≥0.90 |

*Abbreviation:* WHO, World Health Organization.

A recent meta-analysis of published data of 13 studies on the use of FET PET in primary brain tumor including 462 patients showed sensitivity and specificity of 82% (95% confidence interval 74%–88%) and 76% (44%–92%), respectively.[20] Because primary brain tumors are mostly gliomas, sensitivity and specificity were determined as 84% and 62% for the diagnosis of glioma. ROC analysis demonstrated that quantitative analysis using $TBR_{mean}$ and $TBR_{max}$ had a high diagnostic value with respective thresholds of 1.6 or more and 2.1 or more for primary brain tumors and 1.7 or more and 2.1 or more for glioma diagnosis. Moreover, $TBR_{mean}$ and $TBR_{max}$ were significantly lower in grade I–II gliomas as compared with III–IV gliomas ($1.7 \pm 0.7$ vs $2.6 \pm 1.0$, $P<.001$ and $2.2 \pm 0.9$ vs $3.1 \pm 1.1$, $P<.001$, respectively).

Unfortunately, SUV and TBR alone do not allow for accurately classifying glioma on an individual basis, as overlap exists across the different World Health Organization (WHO) grades (Fig. 3). The analysis of time–activity curves allows improving the differentiation between low- and high-grade gliomas (see Box 3). Early ($\leq$15 minutes) maximal uptake followed by a decreasing curve has been related to high-grade glioma (Fig. 4), and late (>15 minutes) maximal uptake followed by a cumulative curve has been related to low-grade tumor (Fig. 5).[12,21,22]

Using a simple index measured in the tumor, the early-to-middle $SUV_{max}$ ratio (e-m ratio = $SUV_{5-10\ min}/SUV_{30-35\ min}$), Calcagani and colleagues[22] showed a diagnostic accuracy of 94% (sensitivity, 93%; specificity, 94%) in differentiating low-grade

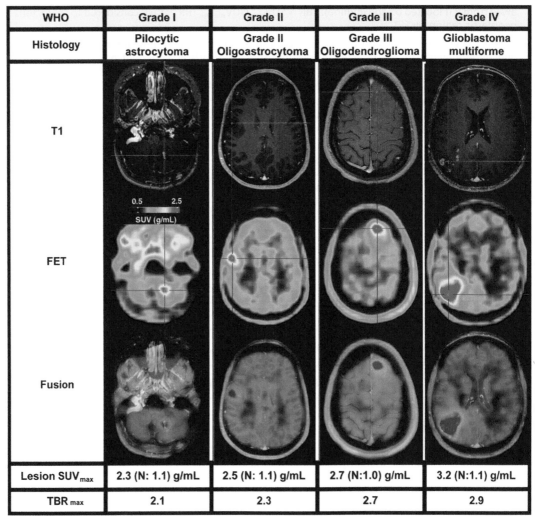

| WHO | Grade I | Grade II | Grade III | Grade IV |
|---|---|---|---|---|
| Histology | Pilocytic astrocytoma | Grade II Oligoastrocytoma | Grade III Oligodendroglioma | Glioblastoma multiforme |
| T1 | | | | |
| FET | | | | |
| Fusion | | | | |
| Lesion $SUV_{max}$ | 2.3 (N: 1.1) g/mL | 2.5 (N: 1.1) g/mL | 2.7 (N:1.0) g/mL | 3.2 (N:1.1) g/mL |
| $TBR_{max}$ | 2.1 | 2.3 | 2.7 | 2.9 |

Fig. 3. Comparison of T1-weighted MR, PET FET, and PET–MR fusion images of WHO grade I–IV gliomas, with the $SUV_{max}$ in tumor and in normal background (N), as well as the corresponding tumor-to-background ($TBR_{max}$) ratio.

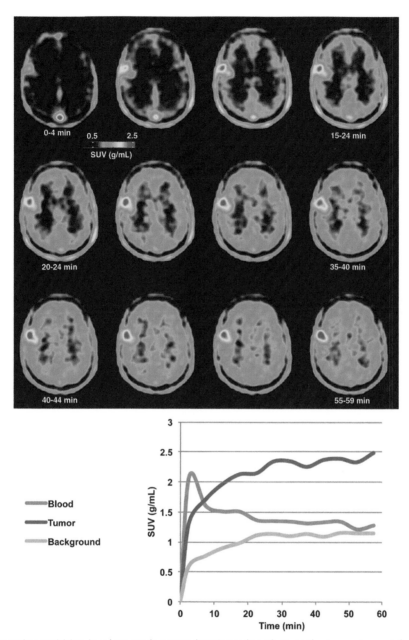

**Fig. 4.** FET dynamic acquisition in a low-grade tumor (WHO grade I–II). Note the increasing uptake in the tumor on the time–activity curve ($SUV_{max}$ tumor-to-background ratio $TBR_{max}$ = 2.1).

(e-m ratio <0.90) from high-grade gliomas (e-m ratio ≥0.90) in a group of 32 patients (see **Box 3**).

Combining FET PET and MR imaging yields good results for the diagnosis of brain tumor. Pauleit and colleagues[23] reported that PET–MR imaging fusion to guide diagnostic biopsy increased specificity from 53% for MR imaging alone to 94%. Similarly, Floeth and colleagues[24] reported that the combination of MR with FET PET and MR spectroscopy yielded a diagnostic accuracy of 97%, confirming the advantage of

a multimodality approach over a single modality one (**Fig. 6**).

## Pitfalls and Variants

For the interpretation of FET PET (**Box 4**), nuclear medicine physicians must be aware of several pitfalls and variants. Increased FET uptake has been reported in several physiologic and pathologic settings: cortical ischemia,[25,26] sarcoidosis,[27] hematoma,[28,29] and abscess,[29,30] often with a low

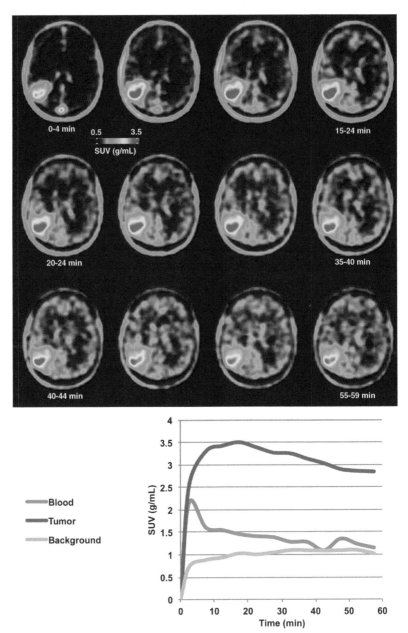

**Fig. 5.** FET dynamic acquisition in a high-grade tumor (WHO grade III–IV). In contrast to the low-grade tumor (see Fig. 4), the FET uptake reaches a maximum before decreasing after 20 minutes (tumor-to-background ratio $TBR_{max}$ = 3.7 at 10 minutes, 2.7 at 55 minutes).

$SUV_{max}$ and TBR, however. Nevertheless, caution should be taken when interpreting FET PET. Because metastases may also have high FET uptake,[31] knowledge of the patient's oncological history and symptoms is indispensable when interpreting images. Finally, because FET presents a high level of vascular uptake initially, vascular lesions may lead to FET PET misinterpretation because of slower tracer washout and inherently

higher uptake than in normal brain (see **Box 4; Fig. 7**).[15,32]

## High-Grade Transformation in Low-Grade Glioma

Histologic diagnosis is based on the most malignant area of the tumor; however, this cannot easily be determined by MR imaging. Preoperative

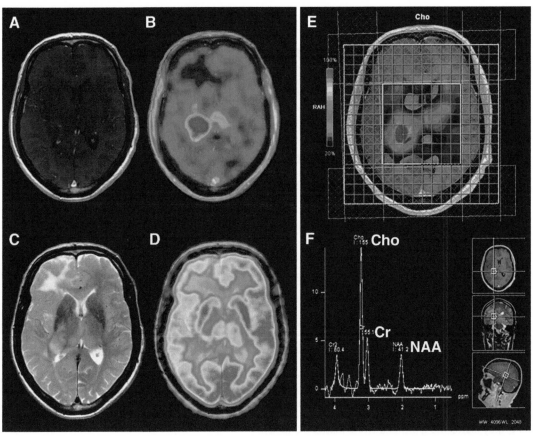

Fig. 6. Anaplastic oligoastrocytoma WHO grade III illustrating multimodality imaging to characterize and delineate tumor. (A) Poor enhancement of the lesion on gadolinium T1-weighted MR images. (B) High lesion uptake on FET PET (SUV$_{max}$ = 2.7 g/mL). (C) Hypersignal of right thalamus and posterior limb of the internal capsule extending beyond FET uptake area on T2-weighted MR image. (D) Low lesion uptake on FDG PET images. (E) High concentration of choline on multivoxel MR spectroscopy. (F) Tumoral spectrum on monovoxel MR spectroscopy with choline/creatine ratio of 2.8 and decreased N-acetylaspartate (NAA).

---

**Box 4**
**Pitfalls and variants**

*FET-positive Lesions*
*Tumoral lesion*

| | |
|---|---|
| Glioma | Teratoma |
| Lymphoma | Medulloblastoma |
| Metastasis | Pinealoblastoma |
| Hemangioblastoma | Primitive neuroectodermal tumor |
| Cavernoma | |
| Germinoma | |

*Nontumoral lesion*

| | |
|---|---|
| Abcess | Astrogliosis |
| Hematoma | Radiation necrosis (Fig. 8) |
| Sarcoidosis | Demyelinating disease |
| Cortical ischemia | Meningioma |
| Aneurysm, telangiectasia and venous ectasia (see Fig. 7) | Pituitary adenoma |

*FET-negative Lesions*

- On FET PET, 20% to 30% of untreated low-grade glioma do not present significant uptake (Fig. 9A); however, when recurring after treatment, this is very rare (see Fig. 9B, C)

- Sequel from ischemic lesion may not show any FET uptake (Fig. 10)

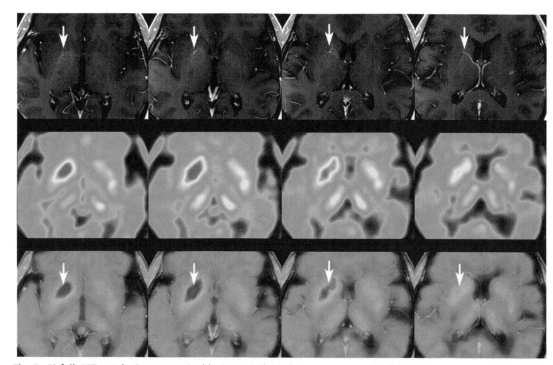

**Fig. 7.** Pitfall: FET uptake in a putaminal lesion, attributed to venous ectasia of the right putamen visible on the T1-weighted gadolinium-enhanced MR image (arrow, $SUV_{max}$ right putamen 2.0 g/mL, contralateral putamen 1.5 g/mL, gray matter 1.3 g/mL, and white matter 1.0 g/mL).

imaging with FET PET allows for directing the biopsy to the area of the highest activity and thus increasing the chances of obtaining a representative tumor tissue biopsy. FET PET dynamic analysis demonstrated high sensitivity in diagnosing high-grade glioma in cases in which MR imaging suspected low-grade glioma.[21] Kunz and colleagues[33] also demonstrated that hot spots in dynamic FET PET could accurately identify malignant anaplastic foci in low-grade WHO II gliomas. Indeed, about 50% of the tumors initially suspected of grade WHO II exhibited grade III–IV PET kinetic uptake.

## Progression versus Pseudoprogression

Treatment of primary brain tumors often involves surgery followed by chemoradiation or radiation therapy alone. Although treatment improves patient survival, patients are rarely cured, and brain tumors frequently relapse. Posttherapy recurrence may be difficult to diagnose and may need biopsy because of poor sensitivity and specificity for morphologic imaging. One of the major limitations of MR imaging is its poor specificity to differentiate between recurrence and pseudoprogression or radionecrosis, which present as abnormalities on T2-weighted imaging

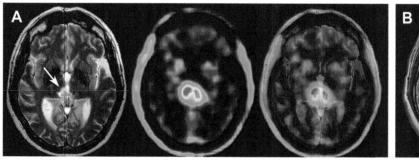
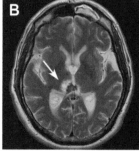

**Fig. 8.** Pitfall: (A) Abnormally increased FET uptake in a lesion post–radiation therapy for a pineal gland tumor. This finding was attributed to radiation necrosis (arrow, lesion $SUV_{max}$ 2.5 g/mL, background 1.1 g/mL, and lesion-to-background ratio = 2.3). (B) This finding was confirmed by stable evolution in size on subsequent 4-year follow-up.

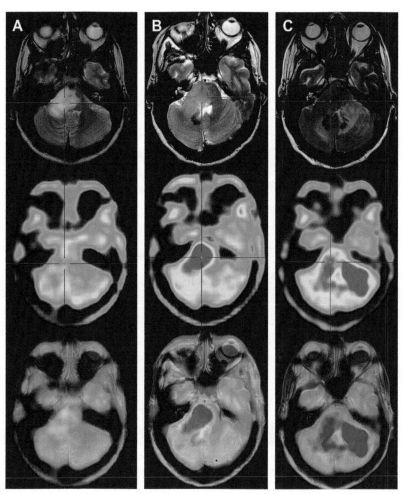

Fig. 9. Typical low-grade glioma on MR imaging known for the past 5 years (unbiopsied). (A) No significant FET uptake is observed, which is a known pitfall in 20% to 30% of low-grade glioma[19] ($SUV_{max}$ lesion 1.4 g/mL, background 1.2 g/mL, and $TBR_{max}$ = 1.2). (B) Follow-up study 2 years after radiation therapy and temozolomide showing a transformation into higher-grade tumor ($SUV_{max}$ lesion 2.4 g/mL, background 1.2 g/mL, $TBR_{max}$ = 2.0). (C) Follow-up after 1 year of temozolomide showing progression with FET uptake in new ipsilateral and contralateral cerebellar lesions ($SUV_{max}$ lesion 3.9 g/mL, background 1.2 g/mL, and $TBR_{max}$ = 3.2).

with or without enhancement on gadolinium T1-weighted imaging. Because FET is taken up more avidly by tumor cells than by inflammatory cells, FET PET could distinguish between recurrence and radionecrosis in rats[34] and in patients with glioma with radionecrosis presenting low $SUV_{max}$ and TBR.[6] Because FET uptake in ischemic lesions is not due to macrophage accumulation but to astrogliosis,[25,26] increased FET uptake has, however, been reported in postradiotherapy lesions[35] (Pitfalls: see Fig. 8). As for the diagnosis of primary brain tumor, time–activity-curve analysis allows one to accurately distinguishing between postradiotherapy changes and recurrence.[35]

FET PET was proved to be efficient in identifying glioma recurrence after initial treatment of low- or high-grade glioma (Figs. 11 and 12).[36] Mehrkens and colleagues[37] reported that FET PET positive predictive value was 84% ($n$ = 24/31 patients) with MR imaging–based suspicion of a glioma progression or relapse as compared with the gold standard using histopathologic biopsies. Rachinger and colleagues[38] reported similar sensitivities for tumor recurrence diagnosis in a series of 45 patients using FET PET as compared with MR imaging (92.9% vs 93.5%), but a better specificity (100% vs 50%). $TBR_{max}$ analysis allowed the differentiation between progression and pseudoprogression pattern, whereas Pöpperl and

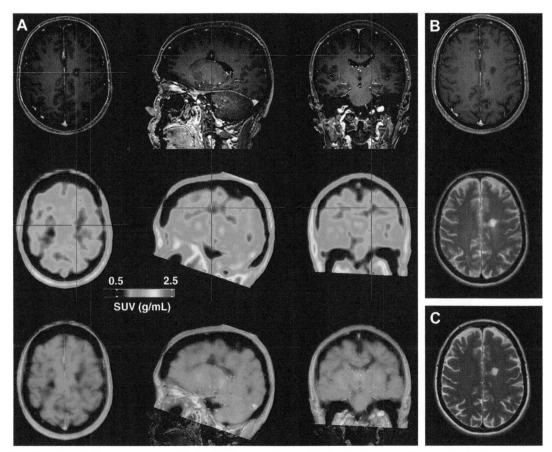

**Fig. 10.** Pitfall: lesion without significant FET uptake. (*A*) No FET uptake is seen in the location of the lesion on T1-weighted and (*B*) T2-weighted MR sequences. (*C*) A control MR image shows no significant change over a 15-month period. The most likely diagnosis was a sequel from an ischemic lesion.

colleagues[35] demonstrated that time–activity curves could differentiate low-grade versus high-grade recurrent gliomas with high sensitivity and specificity (92% each).

### Assessment of Treatment Response

As outlined earlier, FET PET allows for the assessment of residual tumor after the initial surgery.[39–41] After confirmation of recurrence, FET PET remains

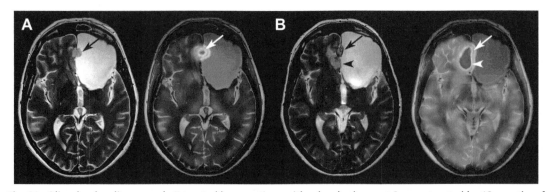

**Fig. 11.** Oligodendroglioma grade II treated by resection, with a local relapse at 3 years treated by 12 months of temozolomide. (*A*) Focal FET uptake (*arrow*) with a $SUV_{max} = 6.1$ g/mL, which was included as biologic tumor volume for radiosurgery. (*B*) Progression at 22 months from the radiosurgery, with a new focal lesion (arrowhead, $SUV_{max} = 7.3$ g/mL) in favor of progressive disease rather than radiation necrosis.

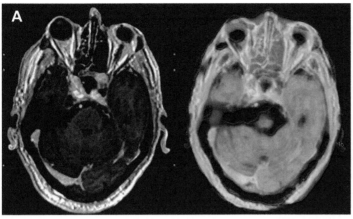
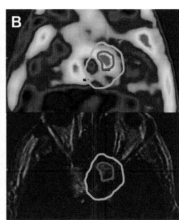

Fig. 12. (*A*) FET PET imaging used for (*B*) radiation therapy planning of a pituitary tumor recurrence with a gamma-knife.

a valuable method to monitor response to salvage therapy by paclitaxel and to distinguish between residual tumor and tumor response better than MR imaging (see Fig. 9).[42] FET PET allows the assessment of early metabolic response to temozolomide in patients with low-grade gliomas, which is correlated with delayed tumor volume reduction on MR images.[41] Finally, after multimodal therapy, FET PET was still proved to be efficient in monitoring the effect of locoregional radioimmunotherapy in patients with grade III–IV gliomas.[43]

## Prognostic Value of FET PET

Floeth and colleagues[44] demonstrated that initial $TBR_{mean}$ on FET PET and diffuse pattern on MR images in untreated low-grade gliomas predicted time to progression and time to malignant transformation. The FET uptake pattern of nonspecific incidental brain lesion was also demonstrated to be of predictive value.[45] A low FET uptake predicted a benign course or the development of low-grade glioma, whereas a high FET uptake predicted development of a high-grade glioma.

FET allows delineating residual tumor volume after surgery and has a strong prognostic impact on progression-free and overall survivals.[39] Postoperative FET $TBR_{mean}$ and $TBR_{max}$ were predictive of disease-free survival in patients with glioblastoma undergoing chemoradiation.[40] Moreover, Galldiks and colleagues[46] showed that 7 to 10 days after completion of chemoradiation with temozolomide, a decrease in both $TBR_{max}$ and $TBR_{mean}$ of 10% or more independently predicted progression-free and overall survival, whereas MR imaging at this early time point had no prognostic value. Finally, after antiangiogenic therapy by irinotecan-bevacizumab, survival was significantly higher in patients with posttherapy decreased FET uptake.[47]

---

**Box 5**
**What the referring physician needs to know about FET PET**

- Why FET PET? It has an increasing role to play in assisting neuro-oncologists and neurosurgeons for decision making in clinical practice (eg, biopsy or extent of resection planning, radiation planning, early response evaluation).

- What to tell the patient about FET PET? Total examination time about 1.5 to 2 hours in nuclear medicine (about 40–50 minutes in the PET scanner); fasting for more than 4 hours before PET is needed, but drinking 1 L water is recommended; no need for glucose restriction or stop of medication.

- Need for correlative MR imaging? Recent (<2 weeks) morphologic imaging with MR is highly desirable; integrative readout between neuroradiologists and nuclear medicine physicians recommended.

- High value of FET PET in non–contrast-enhancing brain tumor on MR imaging, as this does not equate to low-grade glioma. A biopsy-based diagnosis is crucial for the most appropriate treatment. PET helps considerably, as about half of the tumors initially suspected of grade II exhibit grade III–IV PET kinetic uptake. This finding decreases the risk of undertreating such patients.

- PET can affect clinical management in half the patients (mostly from watchful waiting to treat now); whether this will be translated to better patient survival remains to be evaluated.

## Future

Although the European Association of Nuclear Medicine guidelines on PET imaging with amino acids have been published in 2006[10] and allowed for some acquisition protocol standardization, more work is needed for developing criteria to analyze dynamic sequences for tumor grade estimation.

Cost-effectiveness in the use of amino acid PET in addition to MR imaging as compared with MR imaging alone has been investigated by Heinzel and colleagues[48] for guiding surgical resection of high-grade glioma and for guiding targeted biopsy for the diagnosis of glioma.[49] Both studies were based on a probabilistic analysis with Monte Carlo and concluded that, for these 2 indications, the use of FET PET may lead to improved diagnostic accuracy, allowing for improved individual treatment recommendations and outcome in a cost-effective manner. They recommended that more studies including randomized controlled trials are needed.

Finally, amino acid PET changed clinical management in 50% of the patients in a 2010 study[50] (mostly from "watchful waiting" to "treat now"); whether this will be translated to better patient survival remains to be evaluated.

## SUMMARY

Morphologic imaging with MR is the mainstay in the diagnosis and follow-up of primary brain tumor and gliomas. However, it has limited ability to differentiate tumor from edema, necrosis, or fibrosis. PET with amino acid such as FET PET is a promising and complementary diagnostic and prognostic tool to probe tumor biology in vivo. This technique has been used at diagnosis to delineate tumor and estimate its grade (low grade vs high grade). FET PET can be used for planning therapy and allows early detection of residual or recurrent tumor. FET PET helps selecting the site for biopsy in non–contrast-enhancing tumors, which can frequently exhibit higher grade III–IV, decreasing the probability of undertreating such patients. FET PET also changes clinical management in up to 1 patient in 2, most often from watchful waiting to treat now. Pitfalls in FET PET exist, which must be known to obtain a correct diagnosis. Interpretation should be jointly performed with an experienced neuroradiologist. FET PET is of some help when the differential diagnosis includes true tumor progression and pseudoprogression. Finally, FET PET helps in assessing treatment response early and is of prognostic value (Box 5).

Controlled studies on patient-related outcomes such as increase in quality of life and survival, as well as on cost-efficiency, are needed to definitively establish this valuable tool in daily routine diagnostics and management of primary brain tumors.

## REFERENCES

1. CBTRUS Statistical Report: Primary brain and central nervous system tumors diagnosed in the United States in 2004-2008 (Revised March 23, 2012). Source: Central Brain Tumor Registry of the United States, Hindale (IL). Available at: http://www.cbtrus.org. Accessed October 15, 2012.
2. Wester HJ, Herz M, Weber W, et al. Synthesis and radiopharmacology of O-(2-[18F]fluoroethyl)-L-tyrosine for tumor imaging. J Nucl Med 1999;40:205–12.
3. Fueger BJ, Czernin J, Cloughesy T, et al. Correlation of 6-18F-fluoro-L-dopa PET uptake with proliferation and tumor grade in newly diagnosed and recurrent gliomas. J Nucl Med 2010;51:1532–8.
4. Heiss P, Mayer S, Herz M, et al. Investigation of transport mechanism and uptake kinetics of O-(2-[18F]fluoroethyl)-L-tyrosine in vitro and in vivo. J Nucl Med 1999;40:1367–73.
5. Pauleit D, Floeth F, Herzog H, et al. Whole-body distribution and dosimetry of O-(2-[18F]fluoroethyl)-L-tyrosine. Eur J Nucl Med Mol Imaging 2003;30:519–24.
6. Weber WA, Wester HJ, Grosu AL, et al. O-(2-[18F]fluoroethyl)-L-tyrosine and L-[methyl-11C]methionine uptake in brain tumours: initial results of a comparative study. Eur J Nucl Med 2000;27:542–9.
7. Langen KJ, Jarosch M, Muhlensiepen H, et al. Comparison of fluorotyrosines and methionine uptake in F98 rat gliomas. Nucl Med Biol 2003;30:501–8.
8. Babu E, Kanai Y, Chairoungdua A, et al. Identification of a novel system L amino acid transporter structurally distinct from heterodimeric amino acid transporters. J Biol Chem 2003;278:43838–45.
9. Okubo S, Zhen HN, Kawai N, et al. Correlation of L-methyl-11C-methionine (MET) uptake with L-type amino acid transporter 1 in human gliomas. J Neurooncol 2010;99:217–25.
10. Vander Borght T, Asenbaum S, Bartenstein P, et al. EANM procedure guidelines for brain tumour imaging using labelled amino acid analogues. Eur J Nucl Med Mol Imaging 2006;33:1374–80.
11. Laique S, Egrise D, Monclus M, et al. L-Amino acid load to enhance PET differentiation between tumor and inflammation: an in vitro study on (18)F-FET uptake. Contrast Media Mol Imaging 2006;1:212–20.
12. Popperl G, Kreth FW, Mehrkens JH, et al. FET PET for the evaluation of untreated gliomas: correlation

of FET uptake and uptake kinetics with tumour grading. Eur J Nucl Med Mol Imaging 2007;34: 1933–42.

13. Pauleit D, Floeth F, Tellmann L, et al. Comparison of O-(2-18F-fluoroethyl)-L-tyrosine PET and 3-123I-iodo-alpha-methyl-L-tyrosine SPECT in brain tumors. J Nucl Med 2004;45:374–81.

14. Pichler R, Dunzinger A, Wurm G, et al. Is there a place for FET PET in the initial evaluation of brain lesions with unknown significance? Eur J Nucl Med Mol Imaging 2010;37:1521–8.

15. Weckesser M, Langen KJ, Rickert CH, et al. O-(2-[18F]fluoroethyl)-L-tyrosine PET in the clinical evaluation of primary brain tumours. Eur J Nucl Med Mol Imaging 2005;32:422–9.

16. Lau EW, Drummond KJ, Ware RE, et al. Comparative PET study using F-18 FET and F-18 FDG for the evaluation of patients with suspected brain tumour. J Clin Neurosci 2010;17:43–9.

17. Pauleit D, Stoffels G, Bachofner A, et al. Comparison of (18)F-FET and (18)F-FDG PET in brain tumors. Nucl Med Biol 2009;36:779–87.

18. Jeong SY, Lim SM. Comparison of 3'-deoxy-3'-[(18)F]fluorothymidine PET and O-(2-[(18)F]fluoroethyl)-L-tyrosine PET in patients with newly diagnosed glioma. Nucl Med Biol 2012;39(7):977–81.

19. Roelcke U, Bruehlmeier M, Hefti M, et al. F-18 choline PET does not detect increased metabolism in F-18 fluoroethyltyrosine-negative low-grade gliomas. Clin Nucl Med 2012;37:e1–3.

20. Dunet V, Rossier C, Buck A, et al. Performance of 18F-fluoro-ethyl-tyrosine (18F-FET) PET for the differential diagnosis of primary brain tumor: a systematic review and meta-analysis. J Nucl Med 2012; 53:207–14.

21. Jansen NL, Graute V, Armbruster L, et al. MRI-suspected low-grade glioma: is there a need to perform dynamic FET PET? Eur J Nucl Med Mol Imaging 2012;39:1021–9.

22. Calcagni ML, Galli G, Giordano A, et al. Dynamic O-(2-[18F]fluoroethyl)-L-tyrosine (F-18 FET) PET for glioma grading: assessment of individual probability of malignancy. Clin Nucl Med 2011; 36:841–7.

23. Pauleit D, Floeth F, Hamacher K, et al. O-(2-[18F]fluoroethyl)-L-tyrosine PET combined with MRI improves the diagnostic assessment of cerebral gliomas. Brain 2005;128:678–87.

24. Floeth FW, Pauleit D, Wittsack HJ, et al. Multimodal metabolic imaging of cerebral gliomas: positron emission tomography with [18F]fluoroethyl-L-tyrosine and magnetic resonance spectroscopy. J Neurosurg 2005;102:318–27.

25. Rottenburger C, Doostkam S, Prinz M, et al. Interesting image. Amino acid PET tracer accumulation in cortical ischemia: an interesting case. Clin Nucl Med 2010;35:907–8.

26. Salber D, Stoffels G, Pauleit D, et al. Differential uptake of [18F]FET and [3H]L-methionine in focal cortical ischemia. Nucl Med Biol 2006;33:1029–35.

27. Pichler R, Wurm G, Nussbaumer K, et al. Sarcoidois and radiation-induced astrogliosis causes pitfalls in neuro-oncologic positron emission tomography imaging by O-(2-[18F]fluoroethyl)-L-tyrosine. J Clin Oncol 2010;28:e753–5.

28. Salber D, Stoffels G, Oros-Peusquens AM, et al. Comparison of O-(2-18F-fluoroethyl)-L-tyrosine and L-3H-methionine uptake in cerebral hematomas. J Nucl Med 2010;51:790–7.

29. Floeth FW, Pauleit D, Sabel M, et al. 18F-FET PET differentiation of ring-enhancing brain lesions. J Nucl Med 2006;47:776–82.

30. Salber D, Stoffels G, Pauleit D, et al. Differential uptake of O-(2-18F-fluoroethyl)-L-tyrosine, L-3H-methionine, and 3H-deoxyglucose in brain abscesses. J Nucl Med 2007;48:2056–62.

31. Grosu AL, Weber WA. PET for radiation treatment planning of brain tumours. Radiother Oncol 2010; 96:325–7.

32. Stockhammer F, Prall F, Dunkelmann S, et al. Stereotactic biopsy of a cerebral capillary telangiectasia after a misleading F-18-FET-PET. J Neurol Surg A Cent Eur Neurosurg 2011;72:e34.

33. Kunz M, Thon N, Eigenbrod S, et al. Hot spots in dynamic (18)FET-PET delineate malignant tumor parts within suspected WHO grade II gliomas. Neuro Oncol 2011;13:307–16.

34. Spaeth N, Wyss MT, Weber B, et al. Uptake of 18F-fluorocholine, 18F-fluoroethyl-L-tyrosine, and 18F-FDG in acute cerebral radiation injury in the rat: implications for separation of radiation necrosis from tumor recurrence. J Nucl Med 2004;45: 1931–8.

35. pöpperl G, Kreth FW, Herms J, et al. Analysis of 18F-FET PET for grading of recurrent gliomas: is evaluation of uptake kinetics superior to standard methods? J Nucl Med 2006;47:393–403.

36. Pöpperl G, Gotz C, Rachinger W, et al. Value of O-(2-[18F]fluoroethyl)- L-tyrosine PET for the diagnosis of recurrent glioma. Eur J Nucl Med Mol Imaging 2004;31:1464–70.

37. Mehrkens JH, Popperl G, Rachinger W, et al. The positive predictive value of O-(2-[18F]fluoroethyl)-L-tyrosine (FET) PET in the diagnosis of a glioma recurrence after multimodal treatment. J Neurooncol 2008; 88:27–35.

38. Rachinger W, Goetz C, Popperl G, et al. Positron emission tomography with O-(2-[18F]fluoroethyl)-L-tyrosine versus magnetic resonance imaging in the diagnosis of recurrent gliomas. Neurosurgery 2005;57:505–11 [discussion: 11].

39. Piroth MD, Holy R, Pinkawa M, et al. Prognostic impact of postoperative, pre-irradiation (18)F-fluoroethyl-L-tyrosine uptake in glioblastoma patients

treated with radiochemotherapy. Radiother Oncol 2011;99:218–24.

40. Thiele F, Ehmer J, Piroth MD, et al. The quantification of dynamic FET PET imaging and correlation with the clinical outcome in patients with glioblastoma. Phys Med Biol 2009;54:5525–39.

41. Wyss M, Hofer S, Bruehlmeier M, et al. Early metabolic responses in temozolomide treated low-grade glioma patients. J Neurooncol 2009;95:87–93.

42. Popperl G, Goldbrunner R, Gildehaus FJ, et al. O-(2-[18F]fluoroethyl)-L-tyrosine PET for monitoring the effects of convection-enhanced delivery of paclitaxel in patients with recurrent glioblastoma. Eur J Nucl Med Mol Imaging 2005;32:1018–25.

43. Popperl G, Gotz C, Rachinger W, et al. Serial O-(2-[(18) F]fluoroethyl)-L-tyrosine PET for monitoring the effects of intracavitary radioimmunotherapy in patients with malignant glioma. Eur J Nucl Med Mol Imaging 2006; 33:792–800.

44. Floeth FW, Pauleit D, Sabel M, et al. Prognostic value of O-(2-18F-fluoroethyl)-L-tyrosine PET and MRI in low-grade glioma. J Nucl Med 2007;48:519–27.

45. Floeth FW, Sabel M, Stoffels G, et al. Prognostic value of 18F-fluoroethyl-L-tyrosine PET and MRI in small nonspecific incidental brain lesions. J Nucl Med 2008;49:730–7.

46. Galldiks N, Langen KJ, Holy R, et al. Assessment of treatment response in patients with glioblastoma using O-(2-18F-fluoroethyl)-L-tyrosine PET in comparison to MRI. J Nucl Med 2012;53: 1048–57.

47. Hutterer M, Nowosielski M, Putzer D, et al. O-(2-18F-fluoroethyl)-L-tyrosine PET predicts failure of antiangiogenic treatment in patients with recurrent high-grade glioma. J Nucl Med 2011;52: 856–64.

48. Heinzel A, Stock S, Langen KJ, et al. Cost-effectiveness analysis of amino acid PET-guided surgery for supratentorial high-grade gliomas. J Nucl Med 2012;53:552–8.

49. Heinzel A, Stock S, Langen KJ, et al. Cost-effectiveness analysis of FET PET-guided target selection for the diagnosis of gliomas. Eur J Nucl Med Mol Imaging 2012;39:1089–96.

50. Yamane T, Sakamoto S, Senda M. Clinical impact of (11)C-methionine PET on expected management of patients with brain neoplasm. Eur J Nucl Med Mol Imaging 2010;37:685–90.

# Magnetic Resonance Imaging of Glioma in the Era of Antiangiogenic Therapy

Sarah N. Khan, MD[a], Michael Linetsky, MD[a],
Benjamin M. Ellingson, PhD[a,b,c],
Whitney B. Pope, MD, PhD[a,*]

## KEYWORDS

- Glioblastoma • MR imaging • Response evaluation • Bevacizumab • Glioma • Diffusion • Perfusion
- Spectroscopy

## KEY POINTS

- Anatomic magnetic resonance (MR) imaging is the standard method to assess disease status in patients with glioma.
- Antiangiogenic therapy can make the assessment of tumor burden challenging, owing to "normalization" of the blood-brain barrier, resulting in decreased disease conspicuity due to diminishment of tumor contrast enhancement.
- Based on preliminary data, advanced (physiologic) MR imaging may add value to routine anatomic sequences, but confirmatory standardized studies are necessary before these biomarkers can be reliably implemented in clinical decision making.

## INTRODUCTION

Despite decades of study, glioblastoma (GBM), the most common primary brain tumor in adults, continues to have a dismal prognosis. Median reported survival from the time of diagnosis is slightly more than a year, despite standard triple therapy consisting of surgery, chemotherapy, and radiation.[1] Gliomas tend to be highly vascularized tumors, and multiple angiogenic factors have been identified that promote neovascularity and, presumably, tumor progression, including basic fibroblast growth factor (bFGF),[2] hepatocyte growth factor/scatter factor (HGF/SF),[1] vascular endothelial growth factor (VEGF),[3] neurolipins,[4] angiopoietins,[2,5] and the notch signaling pathway.[6]

Recently angiogenic pathway components have shown promise as treatment targets for GBM. The prototypical antiangiogenic drug, bevacizumab, is a monoclonal antibody that targets VEGF-A[3] and has Food and Drug Administration (FDA) approval for treatment of cancers of the colon, lung, breast, kidneys and, recently, recurrent GBM. Although other antiangiogenic agents are being actively evaluated for efficacy against GBM,[7] bevacizumab alone has FDA approval and is now in widespread use as the second-line agent of choice in the clinical treatment of malignant gliomas. Antiangiogenic agents, as a new class of potentially effective drugs, have led to a re-evaluation of standard response measures for GBM, because of their antipermeability effects

[a] Department of Radiological Sciences, David Geffen School of Medicine, University of California Los Angeles, 757 Westwood Boulevard, Suite 1621E, Los Angeles, CA 90095, USA; [b] Department of Biomedical Physics, David Geffen School of Medicine, University of California Los Angeles, 924 Westwood Boulevard, Suite 615, Los Angeles, CA 90024, USA; [c] Department of Biomedical Engineering, David Geffen School of Medicine, University of California Los Angeles, 924 Westwood Boulevard, Suite 615, Los Angeles, CA 90024, USA
* Corresponding author.
E-mail address: wpope@mednet.ucla.edu

PET Clin 8 (2013) 163–182
http://dx.doi.org/10.1016/j.cpet.2012.09.004
1556-8598/13/$ – see front matter © 2013 Elsevier Inc. All rights reserved.

on tumor vasculature, and have increased the difficulty of providing accurate and reproducible measures of tumor response and growth.

## GLIOMA RESPONSE ASSESSMENT CRITERIA

In 1990, Macdonald and colleagues[8] published criteria for the assessment of treatment response in high-grade gliomas. These criteria were based on an estimate of tumor size obtained by measuring the maximal cross-sectional dimensions of abnormally enhancing tissue on contrast-enhanced computed tomography (CT),[9,10] with consideration also given to corticosteroid use and neurologic status. As magnetic resonance (MR) imaging became more common in the 1980s and 1990s, supplanting CT as the modality of choice for imaging brain tumors, some limitations of the Macdonald criteria became more apparent. For instance, the Macdonald criteria rely on measurements of enhancing tumor only (Fig. 1). However, unlike CT, MR imaging is capable of readily depicting nonenhancing tumor, even in the absence of significant associated mass effect. Further, MR imaging also demonstrates that many GBMs are highly irregular and infiltrative, sometimes with indistinct margins,

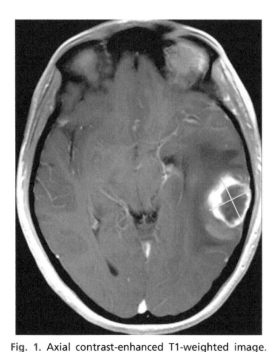

Fig. 1. Axial contrast-enhanced T1-weighted image. The basis for the Macdonald criteria for response assessment in gliomas is the product of perpendicular bidimensional measurements of enhancing tumor. Treatment response is defined as a decrease of at least 50% in the product of the measurements, whereas progression is defined as an increase of at least 25%.

resulting in difficulty in making reproducible bidimensional measurements that accurately reflect tumor size (Fig. 2). Recurrent tumor bordering a resection cavity also does not easily avail itself to reproducible bidimensional measurement. These difficulties are just a few in assessing response in gliomas, not all of which are unique to the Macdonald criteria.

More recent guidelines for tumor assessment, published by the Response Assessment in Neuro-Oncology (RANO) group (Table 1), were developed to address some of the limitations of the Macdonald criteria. The most important difference is that the RANO criteria include the use of T2-weighted or fluid-attenuated inversion recovery (FLAIR) signal hyperintensity as a potential indicator of nonenhancing tumor. The RANO group recognized the difficulty even an experienced interpreter may have in distinguishing nonenhancing tumor from gliosis and/or edema, which also results in increased T2/FLAIR signal, as well as the challenge in accurately measuring regions of T2/FLAIR signal abnormality that may not have clearly definable margins. However, they note that while quantitative assessment of nonenhancing tumor would be desirable, it is currently not feasible with the required degree of reproducibility, and thus a qualitative judgment of a substantial increase in nonenhancing tumor should be considered as tumor progression. The RANO group also addressed 2 other challenges now widely recognized in the neurooncology literature, namely pseudoprogression and pseudoresponse.

### Pseudoprogression

Differentiating tumor progression after radiation therapy from treatment-induced changes remains a challenge. In 20% to 30% of GBM cases, the first MR imaging, typically obtained 4 to 6 weeks after completion of chemoradiation (ie, standard therapy consisting of radiation treatment with concurrent temozolomide), shows increased enhancement that meets standard criteria for progressive disease; however, subsequent scans show stability or even reduction in lesion size, without additional therapy (Fig. 3). This false progression or pseudoprogression is thought to be more common in the era of temozolomide treatment. The mechanism of this increased enhancement that can be mistaken for tumor progression may be secondary to transiently increased tumor and brain vascular permeability effects after irradiation, possibly enhanced by temozolomide, rather than true progression of malignant disease.[11–14] VEGF is

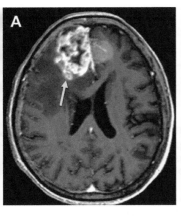 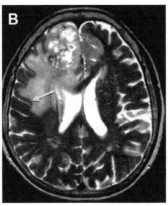

Fig. 2. Glioblastomas are typically avidly enhancing tumors with central areas of nonenhancement representing necrosis. Extensive peritumoral edema is common. (*A*) Contrast-enhanced T1-weighted image showing avid irregular enhancement (*arrow*) with a central area of non-enhancement, presumably tumor necrosis. (*B*) T2-weighted image showing peritumoral white matter edema sparing the cortical ribbon (*arrow*).

thought to mediate at least part of this increased permeability, just as it does in true tumor progression, demonstrating a potential overlap in the underlying molecular changes between these 2 processes that lead to the common imaging findings.

Mischaracterization of pseudoprogression as tumor growth may cause premature discontinuation of effective therapies. In addition, enrolling patients in drug trials that have pseudoprogression rather than true tumor progression could potentially result in spuriously elevated response rates, as subsequent diminution in tumor size would be falsely attributed to drug effect rather than the natural course of pseudoprogression. To address this issue, the RANO group recommends that in the first 12 weeks after chemoradiation, true progression should only be diagnosed if found outside of the radiation field or if confirmed pathologically; however, this stipulation can introduce significant limitations both in the construction of clinical trials and in providing prognostic information to patients.[15]

## Changes in Tumor Imaging Following Bevacizumab Therapy: Pseudoresponse and Nonenhancing Tumor Progression

Marked decreases in the extent and intensity of contrast enhancement may be seen in tumors (in as many as 25%–60% of patients) as early as 1 to 2 days after treatment with VEGF inhibitors (eg, bevacizumab) or VEGF-receptor inhibitors (eg, cediranib).[16–18] This rapid response is thought to be too quick to be attributable to death of tumor cells and shrinkage of tumor bulk. Rather, because GBMs have abnormal vasculature with a blood-brain barrier that is significantly more permeable than normal brain, targeting vascular permeability factors such as VEGF appears

to cause a rapid and substantial decrease in contrast leakage into the tumor, regardless of cytotoxicity on tumor cells (**Fig. 4**). This decoupling of change in enhancing tumor size from antitumor effect can introduce errors in response measures, such as the Macdonald and RANO criteria, that are based on enhancing tumor size. Specifically, reduction in contrast enhancement attributable to reestablishment of the blood-brain barrier rather than tumor shrinkage results in overestimation of response rates to antiangiogenic therapies, and could help explain the discordance between relatively high response rates to these agents with only modest survival benefit (**Fig. 5**).[19]

Another concern with antiangiogenic therapy, in addition to challenges in assessing nonenhancing tumor burden, is whether tumor evades this therapy by invading the surrounding normal brain (**Fig. 6**). Animal studies have identified tumor progression along vascular structures following bevacizumab treatment, so-called vascular cooption.[20] Moreover, some evidence indicates that inhibition of angiogenesis results in increased tumor cell migration.[21] In clinical practice it has been reported that following bevacizumab therapy, patients with malignant gliomas tend to develop diffuse infiltrating disease.[22] This diffuse and infiltrative pattern of disease progression following antiangiogenic treatment has been hypothesized to make recurrent tumor more resistant to additional treatment.[23] To investigate this possibility, the authors characterized several patterns of disease progression following bevacizumab therapy in patients with recurrent malignant glioma[24] including local, distant, multifocal, and diffuse recurrence. Of interest, nonlocal disease is common (nearly 30%) in patients at baseline (before bevacizumab treatment), and most patients do not experience a shift in

**Table 1**
**Summary of Response Assessment in Neuro-Oncology (RANO) criteria**

| Response | Criteria |
|---|---|
| Complete response | All of These Criteria:<br>Complete disappearance of all enhancing measurable/nonmeasurable disease sustained for at least 4 wk<br>No new lesions<br>Stable or improved nonenhancing T2/FLAIR lesions<br>Patients must be off corticosteroids or on physiologic dose<br>Note: patients with nonmeasurable disease cannot have a complete response (stable disease is the best response possible) |
| Partial response | All of These Criteria:<br>≥50% decrease compared with baseline in the sum of products of perpendicular diameters of all measurable enhancing lesions sustained for at least 4 wk<br>No progression of nonmeasurable disease<br>No new lesions<br>Stable or improved nonenhancing T2/FLAIR lesions on same or lower dose of corticosteroids compared with baseline scan<br>Corticosteroid dose at time of scan evaluation should be no greater than the dose at time of baseline scan<br>Stable or improved clinically<br>Note: patients with nonmeasurable disease only cannot have a partial response (stable disease is the best response possible) |
| Stable disease | All of These Criteria:<br>Does not qualify for complete response, partial response, or progression<br>Stable nonenhancing T2/FLAIR lesions on same or lower dose of corticosteroids compared with baseline scan<br>If corticosteroid dose was increased for new symptoms and signs without confirmation of disease progression on neuroimaging and follow-up, and follow-up imaging shows this increase in corticosteroids was required for disease progression, the last scan considered to show stable disease will be the scan obtained when the corticosteroid dose was equivalent to the baseline dose |
| Progression | Any of These Criteria:<br>≥25% increase in the sum of the products of perpendicular diameters of enhancing lesions compared with the smallest tumor measurement obtained either at baseline (if no decrease) or best response, on stable or increasing doses of corticosteroids[a]<br>Significant increase in T2/FLAIR nonenhancing lesion on stable or increasing doses of corticosteroids compared with baseline scan or best response after initiation of therapy[a] not caused by comorbid events (radiation therapy, demyelination, ischemic injury, infection, seizures, postoperative changes, or other treatment effects)<br>Any new lesion<br>Clear clinical deterioration not attributable to other causes apart from the tumor (seizures, medication adverse effects, complications of therapy, cerebrovascular events, infection) or changes in corticosteroid dose<br>Failure to return for evaluation as a result of death or deteriorating condition<br>Clear progression of nonmeasurable disease |

All measurable and nonmeasurable lesions must be assessed using the same techniques as at baseline.
*Abbreviation:* FLAIR, fluid-attenuated inversion recovery.
[a] Stable doses of corticosteroids include patients not on corticosteroids.
*Adapted from* Wen PY, Macdonald DR, Reardon DA, et al. Updated response assessment criteria for high-grade gliomas: Response Assessment in Neuro-Oncology working group. J Clin Oncol 2010;28(11):1963–72.

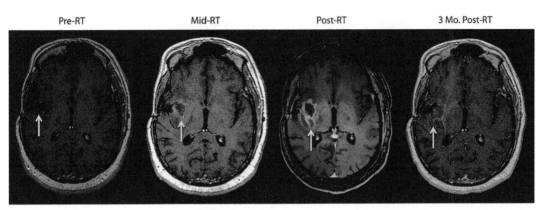

**Fig. 3.** The preradiotherapy (Pre-RT) postcontrast T1-weighted image shows a resection cavity before radiation treatment, with little to no enhancement at the margins of the cavity. During (Mid-RT) and immediately after (Post-RT) the course of radiotherapy, there is a significant increase in the amount of enhancement at the margins of the cavity. The thick irregular enhancing nodules at the anterior margin of the cavity on the Post-RT image are particularly concerning for tumor recurrence. Three months following completion of radiotherapy (3 Mo. Post-RT), enhancement at the resection site has diminished markedly.

tumor pattern at progression following bevacizumab therapy. In addition, patients treated with bevacizumab-containing regimens that progress locally or diffusely have similar efficacy outcomes to one another, including progression-free survival (PFS) and overall survival (OS).

One limitation of earlier studies suggesting more diffusely invasive patterns of tumor recurrence

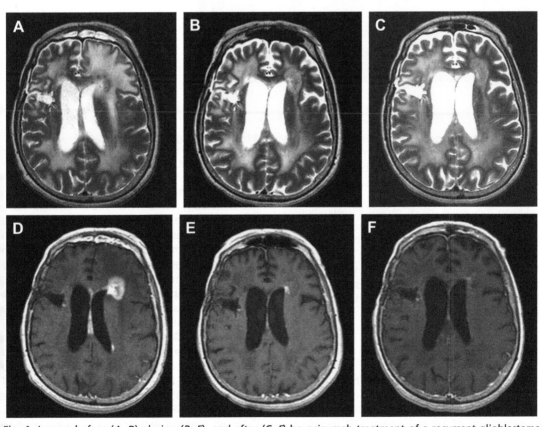

**Fig. 4.** Images before (A, D), during (B, E), and after (C, F) bevacizumab treatment of a recurrent glioblastoma (GBM). There is marked resolution of abnormal enhancement (D–F) as well as decreased edema and mass effect that persisted on additional follow-up imaging. The remaining T2-weighted signal abnormality (A–C) appears mostly secondary to radiation-induced gliosis based on its distribution and lack of mass effect.

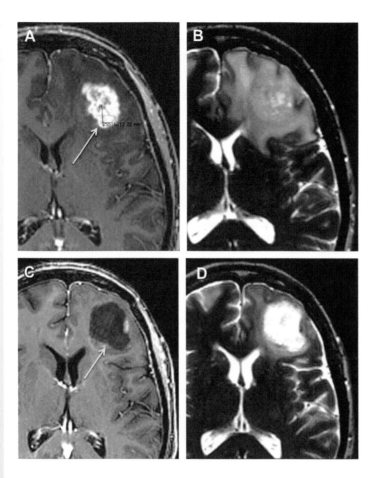

Fig. 5. Baseline T1-weighted postcontrast image (A) showing avid enhancement and T2-weighted image (B) showing extensive edema. The first follow-up after bevacizumab treatment shows near-resolution of enhancement (C, arrow) and diminished surrounding edema on the T2-weighted sequence (D). Although enhancement and edema associated with the tumor have decreased dramatically, the overall size of the lesion is unchanged or even slightly increased. The decoupling of contrast enhancement from tumor treatment response following antiangiogenic therapy has been termed pseudoresponse.

following antiangiogenic therapy is that baseline disease patterns were not noted, making it unclear if patients had diffuse disease before receiving antiangiogenic therapy or if diffuse patterns were an effect of prior treatments. To specifically address this issue, more recent investigations[25] have demonstrated that when compared with baseline disease status, a majority of patients with GBM maintain local disease regardless of multiple recurrences and treatment with bevacizumab, and that survival following progression on bevacizumab does not differ by pattern of disease recurrence (Fig. 7).

## ADVANCED IMAGING TECHNIQUES

Difficulties in distinguishing nonenhancing tumor from gliosis and/or edema and in identifying pseudoresponse and pseudoprogression have led to investigations of several newer MR techniques based on tumor physiology as a way of adding value to standard imaging in the management of patients with glioma.

### Magnetic Resonance Perfusion Imaging

Although more commonly applied for the purpose of stroke imaging, MR perfusion has been investigated as a means of assessing tumors in neurooncology for several years. Groups have investigated the prognostic information available from perfusion imaging and perfusion changes in response to therapy. In particular, perfusion imaging has been considered an ideal modality for the assessment of antiangiogenic treatment, although its ability to serve as a predictive biomarker of response or even an early response measure has been more challenging that originally appreciated. Common methods of perfusion imaging include dynamic susceptibility contrast (DSC) imaging and dynamic contrast-enhanced (DCE) imaging. DSC imaging generates maps of relative cerebral blood volume (rCBV), cerebral blood flow (CBF), and mean transit time (MTT). Dynamic contrast enhancement can be used to measure a parameter known as $K^{trans}$, which is related to the rate at which contrast material flows through blood vessels into the extracellular space

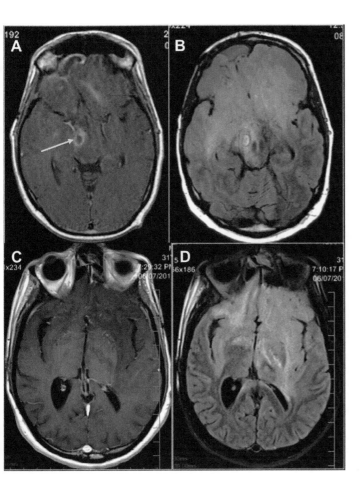

**Fig. 6.** Two cases of extensive infiltrative tumor progression without substantial contrast enhancement in patients with recurrent GBM. A contrast-enhanced T1-weighted image (*A*) shows a ring-enhancing focus near the midbrain (*yellow arrow*) and wispy enhancement in the left orbitofrontal region (*red arrow*), whereas the fluid-attenuated inversion recovery (FLAIR) image (*B*) shows a much larger region of tumor involving both frontal lobes and the right temporal lobe. Similarly, in the bottom row, the contrast-enhanced image (*C*) shows only a few faint foci of enhancement, whereas the FLAIR image (*D*) shows very extensive tumor involving the frontal lobes, temporal lobes, and deep gray nuclei. In both cases, the true extent of tumor is best depicted on the FLAIR images.

as well as the surface area of the capillary bed. In high flow states, $K^{trans}$ can be used as a surrogate measure for vascular permeability.

## Dynamic Susceptibility Contrast Magnetic Resonance Imaging

DSC MR imaging is a perfusion imaging technique that estimates rCBV (**Fig. 8**) and relative cerebral blood flow (rCBF) by using the signal intensity decrease following a gadolinium contrast bolus.[26,27] Specifically, on arrival of contrast in the brain vasculature, T2*-weighted images, which are sensitive to local changes in the magnetic field, show decreased signal intensity in the vicinity of the vasculature caused by dephasing of the blood water spins from magnetic susceptibility differences induced by the gadolinium agent. The T2* signal intensity is then converted to contrast agent concentration using the T2* relaxivity specific to a particular contrast agent.[26,28] Voxel-wise estimates of rCBV are then quantified by calculating the area under the resulting time-concentration curve. This technique, however, assumes an intact blood-brain barrier, which is an assumption typically violated in GBM because neovascularization results in leaky tumor vasculature.[29] To overcome these limitations, experts suggest using a preload of contrast before image acquisition, to partially negate the change in signal owing to leakage of contrast, followed by use of a post hoc voxel-wise leakage-correction algorithm.[30–34]

Neovascularity (angiogenesis) is a defining characteristic of GBM, whereas there is much less vascular proliferation in lower-grade gliomas. Increased vascularity is reflected in increased cerebral blood volume secondary to increased density of capillaries and other small vessels in tumor, and is thought to potentiate malignancy. Therefore it has been hypothesized that increased CBV should correlate with more aggressive tumor, worse outcome measures, and also tumor grade. This hypothesis has been tested in a long-term follow-up study of 49 patients with supratentorial high-grade astrocytoma, in which the

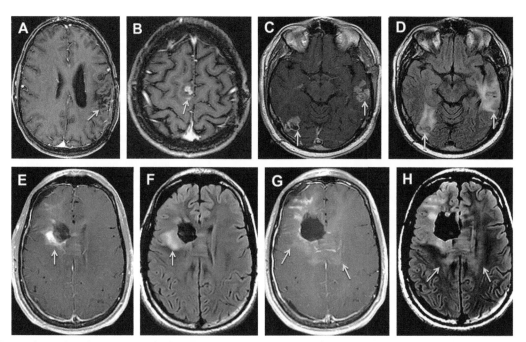

**Fig. 7.** The authors have previously characterized several patterns of progression in recurrent GBM treated with bevacizumab; these include local, distant, multifocal, and diffuse progression. There has been concern that bevacizumab promotes a change from local to diffuse progression, as can be seen in (*E–H*). Distant disease: A T1-weighted postcontrast image (*A*) shows no significant enhancement at the primary tumor site (*arrow*). Another T1-weighted postcontrast image (*B*) shows a well-defined focus of enhancement (*arrow*) distant from the primary site. Multifocal disease: A T1-weighted postcontrast image (*C*) shows 2 well-defined enhancing lesions (*arrows*), with the FLAIR image (*D*) showing surrounding edema (*arrows*); the enhancing lesions are separated by normal signal (*arrows*). Diffuse progression: Postcontrast T1-weighted (*E* and *G*) and FLAIR (*F* and *H*) images show ill-defined extension of tumor (*arrows*) far beyond (>3 cm) the resection cavity margin on the follow-up images (*G* and *H*).

prognostic utility of pretreatment perfusion MR imaging tumor maximum rCBV was evaluated.[35] The investigators found that the maximum rCBV was significantly higher in patients with GBM than in those with grade III tumors (anaplastic astrocytoma), and that this correlated with outcome. Thus the 2-year OS rate was 67% in patients with a low maximum rCBV (<2.0) and only 9% in patients with a high (>2.3) maximum rCBV. Although there is a correlation between tumor grade and rCBV (higher-grade tumors tend to have higher rCBV), measurements of rCBV appear to add value to tumor grade as a predictor of outcome. For instance, Law and colleagues[36] demonstrated that low-grade gliomas with elevated rCBV had PFS indistinguishable from that of high-grade gliomas, because they tend to progress and degenerate into higher-grade tumors more rapidly than tumors with a low rCBV. The investigators reported time to progression (TTP) of 265 days for tumors with initial high rCBV (>1.75), versus TTP of 3585 days for tumors with a low initial rCBV. Mean rCBV values were also determined, as follows: stable disease (2.36 ± 1.78), progressive disease (4.84 ± 3.32), complete response (1.41 ± 0.13), and death (3.82 ± 1.93). Thus elevated rCBV in low-grade gliomas portends a poor prognosis, as tumors with higher rCBV tend to progress more rapidly.

CBV has also been investigated as a marker of response for glioma patients, both for standard (chemoradiotherapy) and antiangiogenic therapy. For instance, changes in rCBV before and 1 month after combined radiation and temozolomide therapy have been investigated as a marker of patient prognosis. In this study Mangla and colleagues[37] found that the percentage change in rCBV after therapy was predictive of OS, with increased rCBV predicting a significantly shorter survival (235 days, compared with 529 days for patients with decreased rCBV).

Several studies have attempted to track changes in perfusion parameters following treatment with antiangiogenic agents to correlate these data with outcomes. In a pilot study of 16 patients with recurrent GBM, Sawlani and colleagues[38] showed that following treatment

Pre-Treatment     Post-Treatment

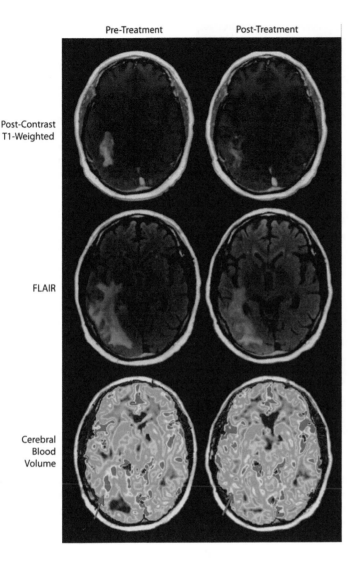

Post-Contrast
T1-Weighted

FLAIR

Cerebral
Blood
Volume

**Fig. 8.** A 61-year-old man with a right-hemisphere glioblastoma treated with bevacizumab after failure of radiation therapy and temozolomide. Following treatment with bevacizumab (right column), there is significantly diminished enhancement, moderately diminished FLAIR signal abnormality, and resolution of the elevated cerebral blood volume (CBV) (*red arrows*) in the posterior cerebrum.

with bevacizumab, tumor hyperperfusion volume (the fraction of tumor with an elevated rCBV) is a predictor of TTP. A multicenter study of 36 patients with malignant gliomas showed that following treatment with cilengitide, another angiogenesis inhibitor, changes in rCBF correlated with both radiographic and clinical response.[39]

Other trials have attempted to use perfusion imaging to differentiate disease progression from pseudoprogression, based on the hypothesis that tumors are relatively better perfused than areas of enhancement that are a result of treatment (radiation) effect. Barajas and colleagues[40] studied 57 GBM patients treated with radiation and concluded that several DSC parameters, including rCBV, were significantly different in patients with radiation necrosis compared with patients with true tumor progression. Thus mean

rCBV was 2.38 for patients with recurrent or residual tumor versus 1.57 for patients with radiation necrosis. Hu and colleagues[41] also demonstrated that rCBV values could differentiate radiation necrosis from tumor recurrence for patients with malignant glioma (both grade III and IV). Image-guided stereotactic biopsy was used to obtain specimens from the margins of enhancing MR lesions (40 samples from 13 tumors), and the rCBV values from the specimen locations were correlated to pathologic analysis. There was a significant difference in rCBV values in specimens diagnosed as tumor (0.55–4.64) compared with those diagnoses as areas of necrosis (0.2–0.71). A threshold value of 0.71 differentiated the 2 groups with a sensitivity of 91.7% and specificity of 100%. It is notable that threshold value for distinguishing tumor from

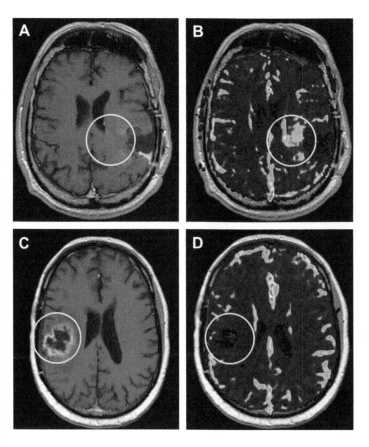

**Fig. 9.** The top row shows a case of true tumor recurrence, wherein the relative CBV (rCBV) is increased (*B*) in the region of faint abnormal enhancement on the postcontrast image. (*A*) In the bottom row, the contrast-enhanced T1-weighted image shows avid irregular enhancement at the margins of a resection cavity (*C*) that would be concerning for tumor progression, whereas the rCBV map (*D*) shows no elevation, consistent with an area of radiation necrosis.

radiation change is quite different between these 2 studies. The threshold and the overall rCBV values in the study by Hu and colleagues were lower than those published by Barajas, potentially related to methodological differences such as CBV normalization (Hu and colleagues normalized to both gray and white matter, Barajas and colleagues to normal-appearing white matter only). In addition, Hu and colleagues included both grade III and IV tumors in their study, whereas Barajas and colleagues restricted the cohort to grade IV tumors.

Sugahara and colleagues[42] performed a similar trial documenting that rCBV ratios of less than 0.6 corresponded to pseudoprogression while ratios of greater than 2.6 represented tumor recurrence, although histologic verification was not available for all of the patients. It is important to consider that regions of enhancement may contain a combination of viable tumor and treatment-related necrosis. Based on this assumption, Gasparetto and colleagues[43] found that an rCBV value of 1.8 distinguished tissue with a threshold of 20% malignant features from specimens with a lesser percentage of malignancy. Another study examined the change in rCBV following treatment

to determine if pseudoprogression could be identified.[37] On evaluating changes in perfusion in glioblastoma patients before and 1 month following chemoradiation, the investigators found that a greater than 5% increase in relative CBV after treatment not only predicted poor survival (median survival, 235 days vs 529 days with decreased relative CBV) but also could be used to differentiate true progression from pseudoprogression. Specifically, they found that patients with pseudoprogression had a 41% mean decrease in rCBV compared with a mean increase of 12% in rCBV for patients with true tumor progression. Taking these findings in composite, it is clear that although the optimal threshold for recurrent tumor has not been established, and there clearly can be overlap between the rCBV for tumor and radiation necrosis, in general, higher rCBV favors tumor (**Fig. 9**).

There are some important technical limitations in the use of gadolinium-based DSC perfusion imaging. One concern in using gadolinium-based agents for perfusion imaging is the leak of gadolinium into the tumor interstitium in regions of abnormal vascularity, which can result in an underestimation of tumor perfusion. Although preloading patients with a small dose of gadolinium before perfusion imaging is acquired, and postprocessing algorithms incorporating leakage correction have mitigated this issue, it would be optimal to have blood pool agents that did not extravasate from the vasculature. Thus some recent work has investigated blood pool contrast agents that stay within the vasculature during the time of perfusion imaging. Many of these agents are based on magnetic nanoparticles, such as small iron oxide particles. A recent pilot study of 14 patients with glioblastoma postirradiation compared DSC perfusion values between a blood pool agent (ferumoxytol) on day 1 and a gadolinium chelate (gadoteridol) on day 2. Ferumxytol-DSC was consistently more accurate in detecting true tumor progression than gadoteridol-DSC, presumably because of the gains in accuracy of measuring rCBV achieved with a nonextravasting contrast agent.[44]

## Dynamic Contrast-Enhanced Magnetic Resonance Imaging

DCE MR imaging is another perfusion imaging technique that uses the T1 relaxation characteristics of gadolinium contrast agents to model the pharmacokinetic distribution of contrast between the vasculature and interstitial space (ie, the Tofts model).[45] Unlike routine contrast-enhanced T1-weighted images, DCE uses serial T1-weighted images acquired during contrast administration to estimate $K^{trans}$, a surrogate for vascular permeability, or the rate at which contrast is extravasating from the intravascular space to the extravascular, extracellular space. (In actuality, $K^{trans}$ is dependent on the product of vascular permeability and vessel surface area, but for high flow states it is a good surrogate of permeability.) Thus, $K^{trans}$ is has been used to evaluate disruption of the blood-brain barrier, which often occurs as a result of neovasculature from angiogenesis (accounting for enhancement of these regions on MR imaging), and is thought to be reversed after administration of antiangiogenic agents.

In one study DCE was used to evaluate 23 patients with high-grade gliomas before irradiation and during the first 2 weeks and second 2 weeks of radiation therapy. Changes in rCBV during radiation treatment were associated with differences in survival. Improved survival was associated with decreases in fractional low-CBV tumor volume at week 1 of radiotherapy compared with baseline and with a decrease in fractional high-CBV tumor volume at week 3 compared with week 1. A smaller baseline FLAIR tumor volume and smaller fractional volume of high-CBV tumor were both also associated with improved survival.[46]

The correlation between clinical outcome and changes in vascular permeability after antiangiogenic treatment has also been investigated. In a trial of 31 patients receiving cedarinib,[47] the combination of $K^{trans}$, microvessel volume, and circulating collagen IV (termed the vascular normalization index) was correlated with OS and PFS. The biomarkers were predictive of a response to cedarinib as early as 1 day after the first dose. In a follow-up study,[48] the same group demonstrated that the vascular normalization index could be simplified so that blood sampling was no longer necessary. The updated DSC MR perfusion acquisition relied on "a novel contrast agent extravasation correction method insensitive to variations in tissue mean transit time." Using this technique, the investigators demonstrated that a higher vascular normalization index value correlated with improved outcomes (PFS and OS) in patients with recurrent glioblastoma treated with cediranib.

Lastly, similar to studies using DSC, DCE also has been used to try to differentiate true progression from pseudoprogression. Bisdas and colleagues[49] recently showed in a study of 18 glioma patients that $K^{trans}$ was significantly higher in the recurrent glioma group than in the radiation necrosis group. A $K^{trans}$ cutoff value higher than 0.19 was highly sensitive and specific (100% and 83%, respectively) for the detection of recurrent gliomas.

## Diffusion Magnetic Resonance Imaging

Diffusion MR imaging has also been investigated as a method to derive biomarkers that can help quantify tumor burden, identify therapeutic response, and predict OS.[50–52] The apparent diffusion coefficient (ADC), a quantitative measure calculated from diffusion imaging that reflects the magnitude of water mobility within tissues, is the most commonly used diffusion parameter for evaluation of brain tumor. Generally speaking, ADC has been shown to be inversely proportional to tumor cell density,[53] although many factors can affect ADC including changes in oxygen tension, blood flow, tissue viscosity, and edema. Lower ADC values correspond to areas of restricted diffusion of water molecules, and thus generally represent areas of greater cell density. Conversely, high ADC values are seen in areas of cell necrosis and edema, where more of the water is located extracellularly and molecular motion is less restricted.[50,54–57]

Given the relationship between cell density and ADC, ADC images (or maps) have been explored as a way to identify and potentially quantify tumor burden. In particular, there has been considerable interest in using ADC or changes in ADC to depict regions of nonenhancing tumor infiltration, especially in the setting of antiangiogenic therapy, in which contrast enhancement is diminished or absent. For instance, Gerstner and colleagues[58] have shown that diffusion imaging can be used to detect nonenhancing tumor in a GBM patient treated with bevacizumab. The same group has investigated the value of diffusion MR imaging in patients with recurrent glioblastoma who received another antiangiogenic agent, cediranib.[59] This study quantified the percentage of peritumoral regions of abnormal FLAIR signal hyperintensity that fell below an ADC value threshold. This analysis showed that these areas of low ADC increased significantly over the course of cediranib treatment "suggesting increasing infiltrative tumor in some patients." The areas of potential tumor infiltration were not visible on contrast-enhanced MR imaging, indicating the potential added value

of diffusion imaging in determining tumor burden. Additional studies will be needed to determine how closely changes in ADC values correlate with increasing tumor density in this clinical setting.

One caveat to this line of investigation is that other processes besides tumor infiltration can lead to decreased ADC. For instance, Rieger and colleagues[60] analyzed 18 patients with recurrent malignant glioma before and after bevacizumab treatment. In 13 of the patients, previously enhancing tumor areas developed infarct-like lesions with decreased ADC. These lesions remained apparent from 4 to 80 weeks, and one such lesion demonstrated atypical necrosis on histologic examination. Similarly, the authors found that malignant glioma patients treated with bevacizumab exhibited persistent diffusion-restricted lesions that were relatively stable over time[61] and did not progress as would be expected for active tumor (Fig. 10). One of these lesions was confirmed to be atypical, gelatinous necrosis

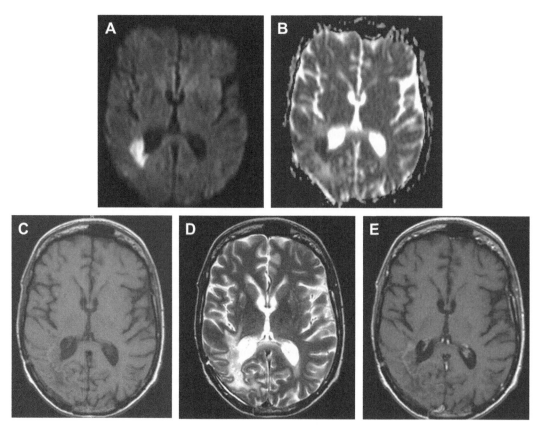

Fig. 10. Development of a diffusion-restricted lesion following treatment of a recurrent glioblastoma with bevacizumab. Diffusion-weighted (A), apparent diffusion coefficient (ADC) map (B), precontrast T1-weighted (C), T2-weighted (D), and postcontrast T1-weighted (E) images. The periventricular location and rim of faint intrinsic T1-weighted hyperintensity are typical of these lesions, which persist and do not seem to represent active tumor. Also, note the lack of contrast enhancement.

following resection. In addition, patients with these low ADC lesions lived longer than patients from a matched control group. Taken together, these data indicate that at least some low ADC lesions in glioma patients treated with antiangiogenic therapy are unlikely to represent areas of tumor infiltration, but indicate nonviable tissue. Potentially it may be possible to differentiate these two processes (tumor vs atypical necrosis) based on absolute ADC values, as the atypical necrotic lesions seem to have lower ADC values than tumor-infiltrated zones, although potentially there is some overlap. In any event, this hypothesis awaits formal testing.

Many studies have used region-of-interest analysis to generate mean ADC values. More recently there has been a shift away from this observer-dependent methodology toward a more inclusive and quantitative approach in which entire regions of brain based on abnormal enhancement or FLAIR signal abnormality are segmented and then mapped to diffusion images with subsequent extraction and analysis of the corresponding ADC values. One approach that has demonstrated utility in this regard is based on the construction of histograms of ADC values from regions of abnormal enhancement (**Fig. 11**). The authors

have used ADC histogram analysis in an attempt to develop a predictive biomarker of bevacizumab treatment susceptibility.[62] In a single-institution study, patients with recurrent glioblastoma in which regions of contrast enhancement corresponded to areas of lower ADC values were more likely to progress by 6 months than in those with higher ADC values when the patients were subsequently treated with bevacizumab. This analysis of ADC from scans before initiation of bevacizumab therapy was more accurate (73% vs 58%) in predicting 6-month PFS than change in enhancing tumor volume at first follow-up, which is the basis for standard response measures (Macdonald and RANO criteria).

To further substantiate the relationship between ADC and bevacizumab treatment susceptibility, the authors retrospectively analyzed data from the multicenter BRAIN study[17] (one of the studies used to gain FDA approval for bevacizumab treatment of recurrent GBM). The ADC histogram analysis was able to stratify not only PFS but also OS for this patient cohort. Thus in patients with low ADC, there was a 2.28-fold reduction in the median TTP and a 1.42-fold decrease in the median OS compared with patients with higher ADC tumoral values. The ability to predict 6-month

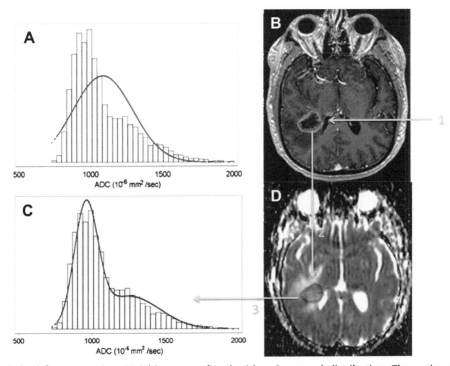

**Fig. 11.** Method for generating ADC histograms fitted with a 2–normal distribution. The entire volume of enhancing tumor is segmented on postcontrast images (1) and overlaid on the ADC map (2). ADC values from enhancing regions are extracted to generate a histogram (3). As the histograms are often bimodal or skewed, a 2–normal distribution provides a better fit than a single Gaussian curve.

PFS was not as accurate as the authors had previously found in their single-institution study. Potentially standardization of diffusion imaging protocols across sites (something that was not done in the BRAIN study), could result in reduced variability in ADC measures, and improved performance of the ADC histogram biomarker.

Another adaptation to diffusion imaging analysis is to assess changes on a voxel-by-voxel level, rather than a change in the mean ADC values in which all voxels are averaged together. This approach has the advantage of maintaining potential differences in treatment response based on spatial heterogeneity in these complex tumors. For instance, it may be the case that a treatment evokes dissimilar effects on different portions of a single tumor. Some areas of tumor could respond to treatment, with increasing ADC values reflecting cell death, whereas other areas of tumor might simultaneously progress, resulting in areas of diminishing ADC values. In analyses of mean change in ADC, these opposite effects could cancel each other out, and thus the impact of treatment would go uncaptured. By using voxel-wise changes in ADC over time, a technique called functional diffusion mapping (fDMs), this pitfall can be circumvented. There is substantial evidence demonstrating the potential utility of fDMs in the evaluation of tumor growth and response to therapy, particularly in GBM where the tumor is spatially and genetically heterogeneous (**Fig. 12**). For instance, in an early fDM study of 34 patients with malignant glioma, diffusion changes at 3 weeks were predictive of radiographic responses seen at 10 weeks.[63] Patients classified as having disease progression by fDM analysis at 3 weeks were found to have a shorter TTP compared with those patients classified as having stable disease (median TTP, 4.3 vs 7.3 months). Thus fDMs may be a valuable early response marker of radiation susceptibility in glioma patients. This hypothesis is supported by a follow-up study from the same group involving fDM analysis of 60 patients with high-grade gliomas.[64] In that report the investigators found that greater therapy-induced increases in diffusion were found in patients alive at the end of 1 year in comparison with those who had died during the same period. Furthermore, the volume of tumor with increased diffusion by 3 weeks was the strongest predictor of patient survival; larger fDM volumes predicted longer median survival (53 vs 11 months). In a much larger study involving 143 newly diagnosed GBMs, the authors examined the utility of fDMs as an early response marker of outcome following radiochemotherapy, generating fDMs from pretreatment and posttreatment examinations. It was found that patients with decreasing ADC in a large volume fraction of pretreatment FLAIR or contrast-enhancing regions had earlier progression and shorter survival than patients with a lower volume fraction (hazard ratio of 3.2).[65] These data support the hypothesis that fDM is a sensitive imaging biomarker for predicting survival in GBM.

The relationship between diffusion imaging and cellularity has been demonstrated in glioma patients using histopathologic analysis. Ellingson and colleagues[53] studied the relation of ADC to cellularity by correlating stereotactic biopsy specimens with ADC maps. ADC was found to be inversely proportional to cell density with a sensitivity of $1.01 \times 10^{-7}$ (mm²/s)/(nuclei/mm²).

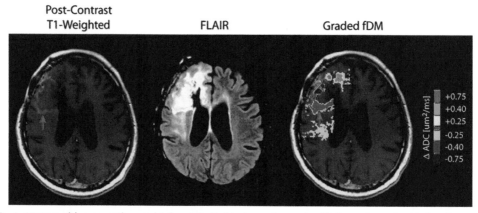

Post-Contrast T1-Weighted    FLAIR    Graded fDM

$\Delta$ ADC [um²/ms]
+0.75
+0.40
+0.25
-0.25
-0.40
-0.75

**Fig. 12.** A 47-year-old man with a right frontal glioblastoma treated with bevacizumab. At the time of these scans, the patient was on bevacizumab. (*Left*) Postcontrast T1-weighted image showing weakly enhancing rim (*arrow*). (*Middle*) FLAIR images showing large extent of possible tumor. (*Right*) Graded functional diffusion maps (fDMs) calculated between the current time point and the previous MR scan session showing regions of relative hypercellularity (*blue*) along the posterior aspect of the contrast-enhancing rim (*arrow*), suggesting this may be the site of growing tumor.

The investigators also performed an examination of the change in ADC that is necessary to classify voxels as significantly increasing, decreasing, or not changing, or in other words, establish a change in ADC from one diffusion image to the next that represents a nonrandom difference attributable to system noise, at the 95% confidence level. It is interesting that this threshold turned out to be tissue dependent: $0.25 \times 10^{-3}$ mm$^2$/s for white matter, $0.31 \times 10^{-3}$ mm$^2$/s for gray matter, and $0.40 \times 10^{-3}$ mm$^2$/s for a mixture of white and gray matter. This groundwork allows the confident assignation of fDM voxels to the appropriate category. Additional work by the same group provided some clinical validation of this principle. In a pilot study the investigators found that in a patient

with gliomatosis cerebri[66] the absolute volume of hypercellularity correlated with a progressive decline in neurologic status, without associated progression of FLAIR signal abnormality or other MR findings. These data suggest that the accumulation of hypercellular voxels by fDM analysis is clinically meaningful, although additional studies are needed to confirm this hypothesis.

Some refinements to the fDM approach appear to further enhance the technique. For instance, "graded" fDMs, in which voxels are categorized not just as increasing or decreasing in ADC but are also analyzed according to the degree of interval change, have been suggested as a possible improvement to standard fDMs. For patients with recurrent GBM treated with bevacizumab therapy,

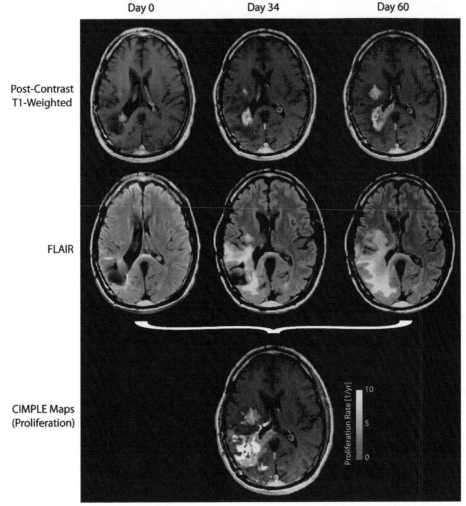

Fig. 13. A 53-year-old man with a left temporal glioblastoma treated with adjuvant temozolomide. (*Top row*) Serial postcontrast T1-weighted images showing tumor growth. (*Middle row*) Serial FLAIR images showing widening extent of the malignant boundary. (*Bottom row*) Cell invasion, motility, and proliferation level estimates (CIMPLE) map estimate of proliferation rate calculated from serial diffusion images over the 60-day time frame.

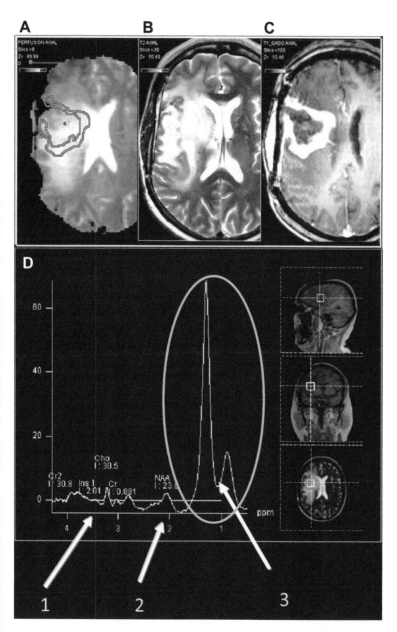

Fig. 14. Spectroscopy provides a noninvasive measure of metabolites. (*Top row*) Dynamic susceptibility contrast (*A*), T2-weighted (*B*), and postcontrast T1-weighted (*C*) images showing an area of possible recurrence at the margin of a resection cavity. Spectroscopy of this area (*D*) shows a low choline peak (*arrow* 1), low NAA peak (*arrow* 2), and elevated lipids/lactate peak (*arrow* 3), consistent with a necrotic area lacking viable tumor. The area of contrast enhancement seen along the margin of the resection cavity is more likely to represent pseudoprogression.

the authors have shown that graded fDMs (showing voxels with decreased ADC between 0.25 and 0.4 $\mu m^2$/ms) are a better predictor of outcome including OS than standard fDMs based on a single threshold.

Another diffusion-based approach showing potential clinical utility is based on mathematical modeling of tumor growth predicated on the assumption that ADC is a direct reflection of tumor cell density.[67] Using serial diffusion data for a given patient, singular values for "cell diffusion rate" and "cell proliferation rate" can be derived to describe growth and invasion of the tumor as a whole. Using

this approach on a voxel-wise basis allows for the computation of an imaging biomarker termed cell invasion, motility, and proliferation level estimates (CIMPLE maps).[67] Because of the known spatial heterogeneity in human GBM, image maps of cell proliferation and invasion calculated from CIMPLE maps may be valuable for isolating the most malignant portions of the tumor, or identifying the portions of the tumor not responding to treatment (**Fig. 13**). In a pilot study,[68] the authors demonstrated the utility of CIMPLE maps to predict PFS and OS in 26 recurrent glioblastoma patients treated with bevacizumab. Voxel-wise estimates of cell proliferation rate predicted areas of subsequently developing contrast enhancement in 35% of patients, and a linear correlation was found between the mean proliferation rate and both PFS and OS.

## Magnetic Resonance Spectroscopy

MR spectroscopy can potentially provide biochemical information that may be beneficial in distinguishing radiation necrosis or treatment effect from tumor recurrence, although evidence garnered to date is highly preliminary (Fig. 14). In MR spectroscopy, the spectral intensity of the major brain metabolites can be overlaid on grayscale MR images to compare changes in adjacent voxels or evaluate the distribution pattern of a particular metabolite in tissue. Ratios of standard brain metabolites, in particular choline, creatinine, and N-acetylaspartate (NAA), have been promulgated for this purpose.[69] In one study of 33 postsurgical primary brain tumor patients examined with MR imaging, new contrast-enhancing lesions were correlated with histopathology and imaging follow-up to establish a final diagnosis of treatment effect versus recurrent tumor. Patients with recurrent tumors demonstrated significant elevations in choline:creatinine and choline:NAA and reduction in NAA:creatinine ratios compared with postradiation change. A predictive model using the choline:NAA ratio had a sensitivity of 85%, specificity of 69.2%, and area under the receiver operating characteristic curve of 0.92.

Another MR spectroscopy–based technique termed 2-dimensional chemical shift imaging (CSI) has also shown promise in differentiating tumor from radiation injury in patients with recurrent contrast-enhancing intracranial lesions.[70] In a study of 29 patients with a contrast-enhancing lesion near a previously treated brain neoplasm, 2-dimensional CSI data were correlated with clinical follow-up, radiographic follow-up, and histopathology. Similar to the above findings, ratios of choline:creatinine and choline:NAA ratios were higher in tumor than in radiation injury, and higher in areas of radiation injury than in normal-appearing white matter. Technical challenges associated with MR spectroscopy, including degradation of images by susceptibility artifact, which is particularly prevalent in posttreatment brains, remains a substantial impediment to its more widespread adoption and validation in larger studies.

## SUMMARY

With the proliferation of new, potentially effective agents in the treatment of malignant gliomas, the search for reliable biomarkers of disease progression and survival has intensified. The clinical utility of the new techniques presented here remains uncertain, as the associated methodology has not been standardized, and early trials have produced sometimes inconsistent results. Among the more promising techniques, the use of ADC histogram analysis has been preliminarily shown to be a predictor of response to bevacizumab treatment, but is currently undergoing validation in larger studies. Perfusion imaging appears to add value to standard imaging in its ability to differentiate true progression from pseudoprogression. Despite the considerable hurdles involved in developing new biomarkers, a reliable way to characterize and categorize gliomas based on physiologic properties and early response to treatment would provide a valuable tool both in the development of new therapies and in the current clinical management of GBM.

## REFERENCES

1. Schmidt NO, Westphal M, Hagel C, et al. Levels of vascular endothelial growth factor, hepatocyte growth factor/scatter factor and basic fibroblast growth factor in human gliomas and their relation to angiogenesis. Int J Cancer 1999;84(1):10–8.
2. Holash J, Maisonpierre PC, Compton D, et al. Vessel cooption, regression, and growth in tumors mediated by angiopoietins and VEGF. Science 1999; 284(5422):1994–8.
3. Plate KH, Breier G, Weich HA, et al. Vascular endothelial growth factor is a potential tumour angiogenesis factor in human gliomas in vivo. Nature 1992; 359(6398):845–8.
4. Soker S, Fidder H, Neufeld G, et al. Characterization of novel vascular endothelial growth factor (VEGF) receptors on tumor cells that bind VEGF165 via its exon 7-encoded domain. J Biol Chem 1996; 271(10):5761–7.
5. Oliner J, Min H, Leal J, et al. Suppression of angiogenesis and tumor growth by selective inhibition of angiopoietin-2. Cancer Cell 2004;6(5):507–16.
6. Kerbel RS. Tumor angiogenesis. N Engl J Med 2008; 358(19):2039–49.
7. Henson JW, Ulmer S, Harris GJ. Brain tumor imaging in clinical trials. AJNR Am J Neuroradiol 2008;29(3): 419–24.
8. Macdonald DR, Cascino TL, Schold SC Jr, et al. Response criteria for phase II studies of supratentorial malignant glioma. J Clin Oncol 1990;8(7):1277–80.
9. WHO. Handbook for reporting results of cancer treatment. Geneva (Switzerland): World Health Organization Offset Publication; 1979. 48.
10. Miller AB, Hoogstraten B, Staquet M, et al. Reporting results of cancer treatment. Cancer 1981;47(1): 207–14.

11. Brandsma D, Stalpers L, Taal W, et al. Clinical features, mechanisms, and management of pseudo-progression in malignant gliomas. Lancet Oncol 2008;9(5):453–61.

12. Chamberlain MC, Glantz MJ, Chalmers L, et al. Early necrosis following concurrent temodar and radio-therapy in patients with glioblastoma. J Neurooncol 2007;82(1):81–3.

13. de Wit MC, de Bruin HG, Eijkenboom W, et al. Imme-diate post-radiotherapy changes in malignant glioma can mimic tumor progression. Neurology 2004;63(3):535–7.

14. Taal W, Brandsma D, de Bruin HG, et al. Incidence of early pseudo-progression in a cohort of malignant glioma patients treated with chemoirradiation with temozolomide. Cancer 2008;113(2):405–10.

15. Wen PY, Macdonald DR, Reardon DA, et al. Up-dated response assessment criteria for high-grade gliomas: Response Assessment In Neuro-Oncology working group. J Clin Oncol 2010; 28(11):1963–72.

16. Batchelor TT, Sorensen AG, di Tomaso E, et al. AZD2171, a pan-VEGF receptor tyrosine kinase inhibitor, normalizes tumor vasculature and allevi-ates edema in glioblastoma patients. Cancer Cell 2007;11(1):83–95.

17. Friedman HS, Prados MD, Wen PY, et al. Bevacizu-mab alone and in combination with irinotecan in recurrent glioblastoma. J Clin Oncol 2009;27(28): 4733–40.

18. Vredenburgh JJ, Desjardins A, Herndon JE 2nd, et al. Bevacizumab plus irinotecan in recurrent glio-blastoma multiforme. J Clin Oncol 2007;25(30): 4722–9.

19. Norden AD, Drappatz J, Muzikansky A, et al. An exploratory survival analysis of anti-angiogenic therapy for recurrent malignant glioma. J Neurooncol 2009;92(2):149–55.

20. de Groot JF, Fuller G, Kumar AJ, et al. Tumor inva-sion after treatment of glioblastoma with bevacizu-mab: radiographic and pathologic correlation in humans and mice. Neuro Oncol 2010;12(3):233–42.

21. Auf G, Jabouille A, Guerit S, et al. Inositol-requiring enzyme 1alpha is a key regulator of angiogenesis and invasion in malignant glioma. Proc Natl Acad Sci U S A 2010;107(35):15553–8.

22. Norden AD, Young GS, Setayesh K, et al. Bevacizu-mab for recurrent malignant gliomas: efficacy, toxicity, and patterns of recurrence. Neurology 2008;70(10):779–87.

23. Claes A, Idema AJ, Wesseling P. Diffuse glioma growth: a guerilla war. Acta Neuropathol 2007; 114(5):443–58.

24. Pope WB, Xia Q, Paton VE, et al. Patterns of progression in patients with recurrent glioblastoma treated with bevacizumab. Neurology 2011;76(5): 432–7.

25. Chamberlain MC. Radiographic patterns of relapse in glioblastoma. J Neurooncol 2011;101(2):319–23.

26. Aronen HJ, Gazit IE, Louis DN, et al. Cerebral blood volume maps of gliomas: comparison with tumor grade and histologic findings. Radiology 1994; 191(1):41–51.

27. Cha S, Knopp EA, Johnson G, et al. Dynamic contrast-enhanced T2-weighted MR imaging of recurrent malignant gliomas treated with thalido-mide and carboplatin. AJNR Am J Neuroradiol 2000;21(5):881–90.

28. Henry RG, Vigneron DB, Fischbein NJ, et al. Comparison of relative cerebral blood volume and proton spectroscopy in patients with treated gliomas. AJNR Am J Neuroradiol 2000;21(2): 357–66.

29. Lupo JM, Cha S, Chang SM, et al. Dynamic susceptibility-weighted perfusion imaging of high-grade gliomas: characterization of spatial heteroge-neity. AJNR Am J Neuroradiol 2005;26(6):1446–54.

30. Boxerman JL, Prah DE, Paulson ES, et al. The role of preload and leakage correction in gadolinium-based cerebral blood volume estimation determined by comparison with MION as a criterion standard. AJNR Am J Neuroradiol 2012;33(6):1081–7.

31. Hu LS, Baxter LC, Pinnaduwage DS, et al. Opti-mized preload leakage-correction methods to improve the diagnostic accuracy of dynamic susceptibility-weighted contrast-enhanced perfu-sion MR imaging in posttreatment gliomas. AJNR Am J Neuroradiol 2010;31(1):40–8.

32. Paulson ES, Schmainda KM. Comparison of dynamic susceptibility-weighted contrast-enhanced MR methods: recommendations for measuring rela-tive cerebral blood volume in brain tumors. Radi-ology 2008;249(2):601–13.

33. Boxerman JL, Schmainda KM, Weisskoff RM. Rela-tive cerebral blood volume maps corrected for contrast agent extravasation significantly correlate with glioma tumor grade, whereas uncorrected maps do not. AJNR Am J Neuroradiol 2006;27(4): 859–67.

34. Quarles CC, Ward BD, Schmainda KM. Improving the reliability of obtaining tumor hemodynamic parameters in the presence of contrast agent extrav-asation. Magn Reson Med 2005;53(6):1307–16.

35. Hirai T, Murakami R, Nakamura H, et al. Prognostic value of perfusion MR imaging of high-grade astro-cytomas: long-term follow-up study. AJNR Am J Neuroradiol 2008;29(8):1505–10.

36. Law M, Young RJ, Babb JS, et al. Gliomas: predict-ing time to progression or survival with cerebral blood volume measurements at dynamic susceptibility-weighted contrast-enhanced perfu-sion MR imaging. Radiology 2008;247(2):490–8.

37. Mangla R, Singh G, Ziegelitz D, et al. Changes in relative cerebral blood volume 1 month after

radiation-temozolomide therapy can help predict overall survival in patients with glioblastoma. Radiology 2010;256(2):575–84.

38. Sawlani RN, Raizer J, Horowitz SW, et al. Glioblastoma: a method for predicting response to antiangiogenic chemotherapy by using MR perfusion imaging—pilot study. Radiology 2010;255(2):622–8.

39. Akella NS, Twieg DB, Mikkelsen T, et al. Assessment of brain tumor angiogenesis inhibitors using perfusion magnetic resonance imaging: quality and analysis results of a phase I trial. J Magn Reson Imaging 2004;20(6):913–22.

40. Barajas RF Jr, Chang JS, Segal MR, et al. Differentiation of recurrent glioblastoma multiforme from radiation necrosis after external beam radiation therapy with dynamic susceptibility-weighted contrast-enhanced perfusion MR imaging. Radiology 2009; 253(2):486–96.

41. Hu LS, Baxter LC, Smith KA, et al. Relative cerebral blood volume values to differentiate high-grade glioma recurrence from posttreatment radiation effect: direct correlation between image-guided tissue histopathology and localized dynamic susceptibility-weighted contrast-enhanced perfusion MR imaging measurements. AJNR Am J Neuroradiol 2009;30(3):552–8.

42. Sugahara T, Korogi Y, Tomiguchi S, et al. Posttherapeutic intraaxial brain tumor: the value of perfusion-sensitive contrast-enhanced MR imaging for differentiating tumor recurrence from nonneoplastic contrast-enhancing tissue. AJNR Am J Neuroradiol 2000;21(5):901–9.

43. Gasparetto EL, Pawlak MA, Patel SH, et al. Posttreatment recurrence of malignant brain neoplasm: accuracy of relative cerebral blood volume fraction in discriminating low from high malignant histologic volume fraction. Radiology 2009;250(3):887–96.

44. Gahramanov S, Raslan AM, Muldoon LL, et al. Potential for differentiation of pseudoprogression from true tumor progression with dynamic susceptibility-weighted contrast-enhanced magnetic resonance imaging using ferumoxytol vs. gadoteridol: a pilot study. Int J Radiat Oncol Biol Phys 2011;79(2):514–23.

45. Tofts PS, Kermode AG. Measurement of the blood-brain barrier permeability and leakage space using dynamic MR imaging. 1. Fundamental concepts. Magn Reson Med 1991;17(2):357–67.

46. Cao Y, Tsien CI, Nagesh V, et al. Survival prediction in high-grade gliomas by MRI perfusion before and during early stage of RT [corrected]. Int J Radiat Oncol Biol Phys 2006;64(3):876–85.

47. Sorensen AG, Batchelor TT, Zhang WT, et al. A "vascular normalization index" as potential mechanistic biomarker to predict survival after a single dose of cediranib in recurrent glioblastoma patients. Cancer Res 2009;69(13):5296–300.

48. Emblem KE, Bjornerud A, Mouridsen K, et al. T(1)- and T(2)(*)-dominant extravasation correction in DSC-MRI: part II-predicting patient outcome after a single dose of cediranib in recurrent glioblastoma patients. J Cereb Blood Flow Metab 2011;31(10):2054–64.

49. Bisdas S, Naegele T, Ritz R, et al. Distinguishing recurrent high-grade gliomas from radiation injury: a pilot study using dynamic contrast-enhanced MR imaging. Acad Radiol 2011;18(5):575–83.

50. Chenevert TL, Stegman LD, Taylor JM, et al. Diffusion magnetic resonance imaging: an early surrogate marker of therapeutic efficacy in brain tumors. J Natl Cancer Inst 2000;92(24):2029–36.

51. Hamstra DA, Lee KC, Tychewicz JM, et al. The use of $^{19}$F spectroscopy and diffusion-weighted MRI to evaluate differences in gene-dependent enzyme prodrug therapies. Mol Ther 2004;10(5):916–28.

52. Hall DE, Moffat BA, Stojanovska J, et al. Therapeutic efficacy of DTI-015 using diffusion magnetic resonance imaging as an early surrogate marker. Clin Cancer Res 2004;10(23):7852–9.

53. Ellingson BM, Malkin MG, Rand SD, et al. Validation of functional diffusion maps (fDMs) as a biomarker for human glioma cellularity. J Magn Reson Imaging 2010;31(3):538–48.

54. Sugahara T, Korogi Y, Kochi M, et al. Usefulness of diffusion-weighted MRI with echo-planar technique in the evaluation of cellularity in gliomas. J Magn Reson Imaging 1999;9(1):53–60.

55. Lyng H, Haraldseth O, Rofstad EK. Measurement of cell density and necrotic fraction in human melanoma xenografts by diffusion weighted magnetic resonance imaging. Magn Reson Med 2000;43(6):828–36.

56. Hayashida Y, Hirai T, Morishita S, et al. Diffusion-weighted imaging of metastatic brain tumors: comparison with histologic type and tumor cellularity. AJNR Am J Neuroradiol 2006; 27(7):1419–25.

57. Manenti G, Di Roma M, Mancino S, et al. Malignant renal neoplasms: correlation between ADC values and cellularity in diffusion weighted magnetic resonance imaging at 3 T. Radiol Med 2008;113(2):199–213 [in English, Italian].

58. Gerstner ER, Frosch MP, Batchelor TT. Diffusion magnetic resonance imaging detects pathologically confirmed, nonenhancing tumor progression in a patient with recurrent glioblastoma receiving bevacizumab. J Clin Oncol 2010;28(6):e91–3.

59. Gerstner ER, Chen PJ, Wen PY, et al. Infiltrative patterns of glioblastoma spread detected via diffusion MRI after treatment with cediranib. Neuro Oncol 2010;12(5):466–72.

60. Rieger J, Bahr O, Muller K, et al. Bevacizumab-induced diffusion-restricted lesions in malignant glioma patients. J Neurooncol 2010;99(1):49–56.

61. Mong S, Ellingson BM, Nghiemphu PL, et al. Persistent diffusion-restricted lesions in bevacizumab-treated malignant gliomas are associated with improved survival compared with matched controls. AJNR Am J Neuroradiol 2012;33(9):1763–70.

62. Pope WB, Kim HJ, Huo J, et al. Recurrent glioblastoma multiforme: ADC histogram analysis predicts response to bevacizumab treatment. Radiology 2009;252(1):182–9.

63. Hamstra DA, Chenevert TL, Moffat BA, et al. Evaluation of the functional diffusion map as an early biomarker of time-to-progression and overall survival in high-grade glioma. Proc Natl Acad Sci U S A 2005;102(46):16759–64.

64. Hamstra DA, Galban CJ, Meyer CR, et al. Functional diffusion map as an early imaging biomarker for high-grade glioma: correlation with conventional radiologic response and overall survival. J Clin Oncol 2008;26(20):3387–94.

65. Ellingson BM, Cloughesy TF, Zaw T, et al. Functional diffusion maps (fDMs) evaluated before and after radiochemotherapy predict progression-free and overall survival in newly diagnosed glioblastoma. Neuro Oncol 2012;14(3):333–43.

66. Ellingson BM, Rand SD, Malkin MG, et al. Utility of functional diffusion maps to monitor a patient diagnosed with gliomatosis cerebri. J Neurooncol 2010; 97(3):419–23.

67. Ellingson BM, LaViolette PS, Rand SD, et al. Spatially quantifying microscopic tumor invasion and proliferation using a voxel-wise solution to a glioma growth model and serial diffusion MRI. Magn Reson Med 2011;65(4):1131–43.

68. Ellingson BM, Cloughesy TF, Lai A, et al. Cell invasion, motility, and proliferation level estimate (CIMPLE) maps derived from serial diffusion MR images in recurrent glioblastoma treated with bevacizumab. J Neurooncol 2011;105(1):91–101.

69. Smith EA, Carlos RC, Junck LR, et al. Developing a clinical decision model: MR spectroscopy to differentiate between recurrent tumor and radiation change in patients with new contrast-enhancing lesions. AJR Am J Roentgenol 2009; 192(2):W45–52.

70. Weybright P, Sundgren PC, Maly P, et al. Differentiation between brain tumor recurrence and radiation injury using MR spectroscopy. AJR Am J Roentgenol 2005;185(6):1471–6.

# Application of Advanced MR Imaging Techniques and the Evolving Role of PET/MR Imaging in Neuro-oncology

Thomas C. Kwee, MD, PhD*, Maarten L. Donswijk, MD

## KEYWORDS

- Brain tumor • Glioma • Astrocytoma • Glioblastoma • MR imaging • PET

## KEY POINTS

- Despite decades of intensive clinical and laboratory research, high-grade gliomas are still considered incurable.
- Noninvasive imaging techniques that improve tumor detection, delineation, and grading, before, during, and after therapy may improve outcome of patients with high-grade gliomas.
- Diffusion-weighted magnetic resonance (MR) imaging (DWI), diffusion-tensor imaging (DTI), perfusion MR imaging, and magnetic resonance spectroscopy (MRS) allow for tumor assessment on a physiologic and metabolic level and can improve several aspects of glioma evaluation.
- Positron emission tomography (PET)/MR imaging is a unique combination of imaging modalities and may contribute substantially to glioma research and clinical care.

## INTRODUCTION

Primary central nervous system tumors arise in approximately 22,910 people and are responsible for an estimated number of 13,700 deaths in the United States annually. They account for 1.4% of all cancers and 2.4% of all cancer-related deaths (excluding basal and squamous cell skin cancers and in situ carcinomas).[1] Gliomas, originating from the support cells of the brain or neuroglia, are the most common type of primary brain tumor in adults. High-grade (World Health Organization [WHO] grade III and IV) astrocytomas are the most common gliomas, with glioblastomas being about 4 times more common than anaplastic astrocytomas.[2,3] This article mainly focuses on high-grade gliomas.

Despite decades of intensive clinical and laboratory research, high-grade gliomas are still considered incurable, with poor median survival (1 year in glioblastomas and 2–3 years in anaplastic astrocytomas).[2,3] A requisite to achieve a better outcome in these patients is the development of noninvasive imaging techniques that improve tumor detection, delineation, and grading, before, during, and after therapy: visualization of the entire tumor and knowing its strengths and weaknesses in the course of time helps optimize therapy planning on an individual patient basis. This optimization, in turn, increases the likelihood of tumor control and minimizes adverse side effects. Imaging may also be used to evaluate the position of the surrounding normal brain tissue relative to the tumor to improve surgical treatment planning

Potential conflicts of interest: None.
Department of Radiology and Nuclear Medicine, University Medical Center Utrecht, Heidelberglaan 100, Utrecht 3584 CX, The Netherlands
* Corresponding author.
E-mail address: thomaskwee@gmail.com

PET Clin 8 (2013) 183–199
http://dx.doi.org/10.1016/j.cpet.2012.09.003
1556-8598/13/$ – see front matter © 2013 Elsevier Inc. All rights reserved.

(eg, separating white matter tracks from tumor) and to evaluate (the effect of therapy on) the condition of normal brain tissue.

Because MR imaging provides high soft-tissue contrast and multiple (anatomic and functional) tissue contrasts, it is frequently used in patients with (suspicion of) high-grade glioma. MR imaging with (contrast-enhanced) T1-weighted, T2-weighted, and fluid-attenuated inversion recovery (FLAIR) sequences has been principally used to identify the tumor, distinguish tumors from other pathologic processes, and depict the basic signs of tumor response to therapy, such as change in size and degree of contrast material enhancement.[4] However, its role in the management of patients with high-grade gliomas needs to be improved. Final diagnosis and tumor grade are based on histopathologic examination of tumor biopsy samples or by surgical resection.[2,3] More accurate prediction of the tumor location with the highest grade could increase the accuracy of obtaining brain biopsies. A factor contributing to the poor survival of patients with high-grade gliomas is the inability of currently available imaging techniques to accurately delineate the tumor, as a result of which targeted focal treatments may not be effective.[2–4] In addition, conventional imaging cannot provide an early assessment of the effectiveness of radiation and/ or chemotherapy.[2–4] Another unsolved issue is the distinction between treatment effects and tumor persistence or recurrence.[2–4]

The arsenal of available MR imaging techniques has expanded over the past few years, going beyond assessment of morphology and gross degree of contrast enhancement to tumor assessment on a physiologic and metabolic level. New methods such as DWI, DTI, perfusion MR imaging, and MRS may improve the evaluation of high-grade gliomas. The combination of these advanced MR imaging techniques with PET using [18]F-fluoro-2-deoxy-D-glucose (FDG) or other non-FDG tracers may further improve diagnostic and prognostic yield.

This article reviews the value of a selection of important advanced MR imaging techniques (DWI, DTI, perfusion MR imaging, and MRS) and the evolving role of PET/MR imaging in the evaluation of high-grade gliomas in various settings. This review introduces the reader to the basic principles and clinical applications of these advanced MR imaging and PET/MR imaging techniques.

# DIFFUSION-WEIGHTED MR IMAGING
## Basic Principles

DWI allows visualization and measurement of the random (Brownian) extracellular, intracellular, and transcellular motion of water molecules, driven by their internal thermal energy.[5] The signal intensity at DWI is a function of the Brownian motion of an ensemble of water molecules.[6] In biologic tissue, the presence of impeding barriers (such as cell membranes, fibers, and macromolecules) interferes with the free displacement (diffusion) of water molecules.[7] Consequently, in biologic tissue, the signal intensity at DWI depends on the separation and permeability of these restricting boundaries. As introduced by Stejskal and Tanner,[8] the most common approach to render MR imaging sensitive to diffusion is to place 2 strong symmetric gradient lobes (diffusion-sensitizing gradients) on either side of the 180° refocusing pulse in a spin-echo sequence. The degree of signal attenuation at DWI depends both on the magnitude of diffusion and the degree of diffusion weighting that is applied. In biologic tissue, diffusion is expressed and quantified by means of an apparent diffusion coefficient (ADC). A pixel-by-pixel map (so-called ADC map), whose intensity yields quantitative estimation of the regional ADC, is obtained by postprocessing. ADC mapping also eliminates any residual T2 signal that is seen on native diffusion-weighted images (DWI is basically a T2-weighted sequence).[6] Measurement of the ADC would be expected to be useful in tumor assessment because variations in water content (and diffusivity), which can be found within tumors for various reasons (eg, necrosis and variations in cellularity) and adjacent to tumors (eg, vasogenic edema), likely provide information that is not readily available from conventional MR imaging.[4] More details on the background of DWI are discussed elsewhere.[9,10]

## Clinical Applications

The utility of ADC measurements for evaluating gliomas preoperatively for histologic grade has been investigated by multiple studies.[4] Although the ADC is generally thought to be inversely correlated with tumor cellularity, and hence tumor grade (ie, high-grade gliomas generally have lower ADCs than low-grade gliomas), its clinical utility remains limited because of substantial overlap in the regional ADCs between gliomas of differing grades.[4,11] Other methods have been explored to improve glioma grading using ADC measurements, such as measuring minimum ADCs (which is based on the assumption that the regions with minimum ADCs reflect the sites of highest cellularity within heterogeneous tumors),[11] assessing intratumoral heterogeneity on ADC maps,[11] and analyzing histograms of ADC maps based on tumor volume data instead of region of interest analysis on a representative section of the tumor,[12] but none of these methods has (consistently) shown to be superior to conventional ADC measurements.

Accurate tumor delineation is important for planning targeted focal treatments. In the case of high-grade gliomas, however, microscopic clusters of such cells have been detected at autopsy at a considerable distance from the primary tumor mass.[4,13] In addition, studies with MRS have shown that, in a substantial number of cases, abnormal spectra consistent with tumor can be seen beyond the contrast-enhancing tumor and regions that are abnormal on T2-weighted images.[4,14] As has already been pointed out by other researchers,[4] current (echo-planar imaging-based) DWI techniques that are characterized by low signal-to-noise ratio and large voxel size are not able to depict such small clusters of neoplastic cells, which may occupy a small fraction of a voxel. In fact, in a study in which ADCs in specific locations were directly correlated to pathologic examination findings of neuronavigated biopsies obtained at those sites, the ADC was found to be not helpful for distinguishing tumor tissue from peritumoral brain tissue in gliomas.[15]

Response to therapy in glioma patients is most frequently assessed using the MacDonald criteria, which are based on 2-dimensional changes in tumor size on contrast-enhanced MR imaging.[16] To more accurately determine the efficacy of conventional and novel therapeutic agents in glioblastoma multiforme, discriminate pseudoprogression (ie, treatment-related reaction of the tumor with an increase in enhancement and/or edema on MR imaging suggestive of tumor progression but without increased tumor activity[17]) from real tumor progression, and discriminate pseudoresponse (ie, decrease in contrast enhancement and/or edema of brain tumors on MR imaging without a true antitumor effect[17]) from true response, new imaging response criteria have been proposed by the Response Assessment in Neuro-Oncology (RANO) Working Group.[18] These criteria take into account changes on FLAIR or T2-weighted images, as well as contrast-enhanced T1-weighted images. However, it remains to be seen whether the RANO criteria will improve the accuracy of the early evaluation of (novel) therapies. Meanwhile, the value of several functional imaging techniques, including DWI, has been evaluated for earlier response assessment (tumor size measurements in general do not allow individualizing treatment, because the measurements are made well after the completion of therapy). DWI may function as a surrogate

marker for both tissue cellularity and response to treatment (responding tumors generally exhibit an increase in ADC) that occur earlier than the usual measures of tumor response.[19] A voxel-based quantitative DWI approach was introduced (parametric response mapping [PRM] of ADC [$PRM_{ADC}$]), which allows visualization and calculation of tumor diffusion coefficient changes during treatment and takes into account spatial heterogeneity of tumor response (unlike mean diffusion coefficient measurements).[20] $PRM_{ADC}$ combined with traditional radiological response criteria proved to provide a significantly better prediction of the response to therapy than traditional radiological criteria or $PRM_{ADC}$ alone.[20] Similar results have been reported by other researchers who included patient populations undergoing antiangiogenic therapies (**Fig. 1**).[21] However, it has also been reported that DWI may not be sufficiently specific to differentiate pseudoprogression from true tumor progression.[22] In addition, further studies on the reproducibility of this method and consensus on standardization regarding data acquisition and analysis are required before it can be implemented in clinical practice.[23]

The distinction between radiation-induced necrosis and tumor recurrence, especially in the delayed setting, by using conventional contrast-enhanced MR imaging has been difficult; both entities typically demonstrate gadolinium enhancement. It is hypothesized that recurrent tumor contains dense glioma cells, which impede water diffusion (ie, low ADC), whereas radiation-induced brain injury mainly consists of necrotic tissue and gliosis with higher water mobility (ie, higher ADC). Although some studies found quantitative DWI with ADC and/or ADC ratio (ie, ratio of ADC of enhancing lesion to ADC of contralateral white matter) measurements to be useful in differentiating radiation effects from tumor recurrence or progression,[24–26] other studies reported that ADC measurements were of no (additional) value in differentiating between tumor recurrence and radiation injury.[27,28]

## DIFFUSION-TENSOR IMAGING
### Basic Principles

Water diffusion parallel to the white matter tracts is less impeded than water diffusion perpendicular to them, a phenomenon termed "diffusion anisotropy."[29] Highly compact white matter tracts exhibit a high degree of anisotropy, and less compact white matter pathways exhibit lesser degrees of anisotropy. All types of white matter typically show greater degrees of anisotropy than are seen in gray matter structures.[29] As such, diffusion

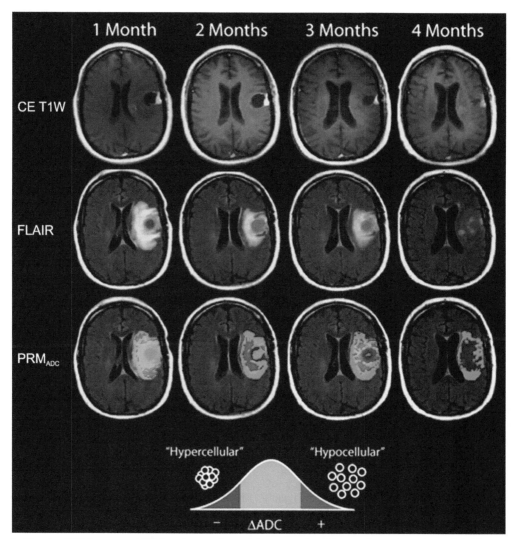

**Fig. 1.** Standard MR image and PRM$_{ADC}$ in a patient with progressive disease after treatment with bevacizumab. A 47-year-old man with a history of glioblastoma multiforme (WHO grade IV) completed radiation therapy with concurrent temozolomide, followed by adjuvant temozolomide. His tumor recurred radiographically just before baseline ADC maps. The patient was then administered bevacizumab monotherapy, and initially contrast enhancement and FLAIR signal abnormality improved substantially. The patient declined neurologically over 4 months of bevacizumab treatment, despite a positive radiographic response on contrast-enhanced T1-weighted (CE T1W, *top row*) and FLAIR images (FLAIR, *middle row*). The patient expired 2 months from the last PRM$_{ADC}$ time point (6 months after start of bevacizumab treatment). During bevacizumab treatment, PRM$_{ADC}$ maps (PRM$_{ADC}$, *lower row*) showed a rapid increase in the volume of hypercellularity, indicating failed treatment. (*Reproduced from* Ellingson BM, Malkin MG, Rand SD, et al. Volumetric analysis of functional diffusion maps is a predictive imaging biomarker for cytotoxic and anti-angiogenic treatments in malignant gliomas. J Neuroon-col 2011;102(1):95–103; with permission.)

anisotropy is used as a marker for white matter tract integrity. DTI is an advanced MR imaging technique that exploits the presence of diffusion anisotropy in white matter tracts to estimate the fiber direction of neural pathways. Typical DTI techniques sample water motion in at least 6 (typical 9, 16, or 32) noncollinear directions (rather than in 3 directions as is usual in conventional DWI), and this allows calculation of a diffusion tensor (a 3 × 3 matrix) for each voxel. This tensor is able to fully describe the molecular mobility along each direction and the correlation between these directions. The entries of the tensor reflect average diffusion and degree of anisotropy in each voxel. It is important to determine the main directions of diffusivities, called eigenvectors, in each voxel, and the diffusion values, called eigenvalues, associated with these directions. The eigenvalues represent the diffusion coefficients in the main directions of diffusivities of the medium. Most common parameters, such as mean diffusivity (an overall measure of the diffusion in a voxel or region), fractional anisotropy (FA, expressed as a ratio between 0 and 1, where complete isotropic diffusivity is 0 and complete anisotropic diffusivity in a single direction is 1), axial diffusivity (the diffusivity along the main axis), and radial diffusivity (the average diffusivity of the 2 minor axes) are derived from them. The reconstruction of nerve fiber tracts of DTI data is called tractography. This technique is based on connecting voxels to build a whole fiber to investigate the fiber architecture in the brain.[9,30] DTI with tractography is useful for providing guidance in neurosurgical procedures by both preoperatively and intraoperatively depicting (the relationship of tumors relative to) important white matter tracts (**Fig. 2**).[31] Details about the theoretical and mathematical underpinnings of DTI are discussed elsewhere.[9,30]

## Clinical Applications

The value of DTI in preoperative grading of gliomas is still controversial. Some investigators reported the FA values of high-grade gliomas to be significantly higher than those of low-grade gliomas.[32,33] The biophysical explanation for the observed difference in FA values between both groups remain unclear.[32,33] Other investigators found no difference in DTI metrics between both the groups.[34,35]

Because high-grade gliomas preferentially infiltrate along white matter tracks, a method like DTI, which can show white matter disruption, may improve tumor delineation and detect occult tumor infiltration. It should be realized, however, that this approach has the disadvantage of indirectly providing information on tumor spread. Some studies have shown that DTI reveals larger

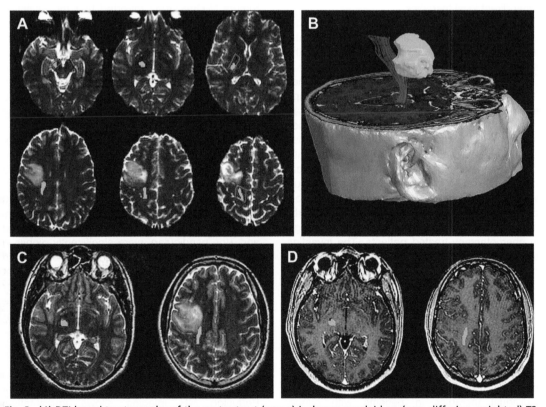

**Fig. 2.** (*A*) DTI-based tractography of the motor tract (*green*) is shown overlaid on (non–diffusion-weighted) T2-weighted echo-planar images. Starting and target regions of interest (*red outlines*) are shown in the cerebral peduncle, posterior limb of the internal capsule, and precentral gyrus. (*B*) The resultant fiber tracks (*red*) are shown adjacent to the tumor (*green*) in 3 dimensions. (*C*) Tractography (*green*) is registered to the T2-weighted and (*D*) contrast-enhanced T1-weighted volumes. (*Reproduced from* Berman J. Diffusion MR tractography as a tool for surgical planning. Magn Reson Imaging Clin N Am 2009;17(2):205–14; with permission.)

peritumoral abnormalities in gliomas that are not apparent on conventional MR imaging, a feature that is absent with minimally or noninfiltrative tumors such as metastases or meningeomas.[36,37] These abnormalities seem to precede the development of gross tumor recurrence on follow-up imaging. Using direct histopathologic correlation, investigators have reported FA and mean diffusivity values to be inversely correlated with the total number of tumor cells and the ratio of tumor to normal cells.[38] In another study that used an analysis method that split the diffusion tensor into pure isotropic and anisotropic components, DTI could correctly identify tumor infiltration with an overall sensitivity of 98% and specificity of 81%.[39] Using this method, it is possible to define a region that corresponds to the tumor margin. A retrospective study suggested that the arrangement of this region could predict the pattern of glioma recurrence.[40] Although these studies suggest that DTI may be of value in delineating the tumor margin in gliomas, further prospective studies are required before this DTI information can be incorporated into radiation therapy planning protocols or help guiding other direct local therapies.

A new concept of using DTI to achieve more individualized therapy has recently been demonstrated in a study in patients with breast cancer.[41] In that study, DTI was performed before the start of chemotherapy (t1) and 3 to 4 months after treatment (t2).[41] In contrast to controls, the chemotherapy-treated group performed significantly worse on attention tests, psychomotor speed, and memory at t2 than at t1. In the chemotherapy-treated group, significant decreases in FA were found in frontal, parietal, and occipital white matter tracts after treatment, whereas for both control groups, FA values were the same between t1 and t2. Furthermore, performance changes in attention and verbal memory correlated with mean regional FA changes in chemotherapy-treated patients. The investigators concluded that their results provided evidence of longitudinal changes in cognitive functioning and cerebral white matter integrity after chemotherapy, as well as an association between both. In addition, longitudinal changes in FA may serve as a neuropathologic biomarker for treatment-induced neurotoxicity.[41] In other words, DTI may have potential in determining patient tolerability to therapeutic interventions such as chemotherapy and radiation therapy. This information may be helpful to tailor individual therapies in patients with cancer, including patients with malignant brain tumors such as high-grade gliomas.

There is little to no data in the literature on the use of DTI for (early) response assessment in glioma. An animal study using a rat brain glioma model reported that as tumors grew in size, significant anisotropy of water diffusion was seen both within and around the tumor.[42] The tissue water surrounding the tumor exhibited high planar anisotropy, as opposed to the linear anisotropy normally seen in white matter, indicating that cells were experiencing stress in a direction normal to the tumor border. When tumors were sufficiently large, significant anisotropy was also seen within the tumor because of longer-range organization of cancer cells within the tumor borders. The investigators of this study concluded that these findings have important implications for DWI experiments examining tumor growth and response to therapy.[42]

It is hypothesized that the normal structure of fibers and cells are usually damaged within astrocytic tumors, and, consequently, the degree of diffusion anisotropy would be decreased (ie, lower FA) than within normal white matter. On the other hand, there are almost no normal fibers and cell structures in areas with the radiation injury, as a result of which the diffusion anisotropy would be decreased (ie, lower FA) than in recurrent tumors.[43] One study reported that the FA value and FA ratio (ie, FA tumor/FA contralateral normal white matter) in recurrent tumors were significantly higher than in areas of radiation injury.[26] Another study reported that, although the FA values in the contrast-enhancing lesions were not significantly different between patients with recurrence and those without recurrence, the FA ratio at the contrast-enhancing lesion area was found to be significantly higher in patients with recurrent tumor compared with those with radiation injury.[25] In addition, both eigenvalue indices, λ(parallel) and λ(perpendicular), were significantly higher in contrast-enhancing lesions in the recurrence group than in those in the nonrecurrence group. In addition, both eigenvalue indices, λ(parallel) and λ(perpendicular), were significantly higher in perilesional edema than in normal white matter in both groups.[25] Despite the reported significant differences in DTI parameters between tumor recurrence and radiation injury by retrospective studies,[25,26] the diagnostic value of DTI in discriminating the 2 entities remains unknown.

## PERFUSION MR IMAGING
### Basic Principles

Perfusion MR imaging allows (quantitative) assessment of the functional aspects of tumor neovascularity in vivo.[44–46] In this section, perfusion MR imaging using exogenous contrast agents (later on simply referred to as "perfusion MR imaging") is discussed; techniques that are based on endogenous contrast mechanisms such as arterial spin labeling and blood oxygenation level–dependent imaging are not addressed. Perfusion MR imaging is performed by obtaining sequential MR scans before, during, and after the injection of a contrast agent (most often a low-molecular-weight gadolinium-containing compound such as gadopentetate dimeglumine).[44–46] Perfusion MR imaging is performed using dynamic T2*-weighted or T1-weighted methods. Dynamic T2*-weighted or suscepti-bility-weighted methods (ie, dynamic contrast-enhanced susceptibility-weighted [DSC] MR imaging) take advantage of the fact that the first pass of a contrast agent through a tissue causes a transient signal drop due to the local magnetic susceptibility (T2*) effects of the contrast agent. The changes in signal intensity are characterized by parameters such as mean transit time, relative blood volume (rCBV), and relative blood flow (rCBF). Dynamic T2*-weighted methods provide information about tumor perfusion, which may be related pathologically to tumor grade and vessel density.[4–46] Dynamic T1-weighted methods (by default, this technique is referred to as dynamic contrast-enhanced [DCE] MR imaging), on the other hand, take advantage of the T1-shortening effects of the contrast agent that cause an increase in signal intensity as it passes from the blood into the extracellular space of tissues. Different models have been proposed to analyze changes in the signal intensity and calculate parameters such as fractional blood volume and permeability metrics such as $K^{trans}$ (volume transfer constant between the blood plasma and extravascular extracellular space), $k_{ep}$ (rate constant between the extravascular extracellular space and blood plasma), and $v_e$ (volume of extravascular extracellular space per unit volume of tissue). Dynamic T1 methods can provide information about blood vessel permeability, capillary surface area, and leakage space, which may be related pathologically to tumor grade, microvessel density, and levels of vascular endothelial growth factor expression.[44–46] More details on the background of perfusion MR imaging are discussed elsewhere.[44,45]

## Clinical Applications

DSC-MR imaging has the capability not only of differentiating low- from high-grade gliomas but also of predicting progression and survival.[47] High-grade gliomas generally have higher rCBV than low-grade gliomas (**Fig. 3**), and it has been reported that rCBV can increase the sensitivity and positive predictive value when compared with conventional MR imaging alone in determining tumor grade.[48] It has also been reported that this method can be used to predict median time to progression in patients with gliomas, independent of pathologic findings; patients who have high-grade gliomas and low-grade gliomas with a high rCBV (>1.75) have a significantly more rapid time to progression than do patients who have gliomas with a low rCBV.[49] With further optimization and improvements to automate postprocessing and quantification techniques, the rCBV measurement may provide an important imaging biomarker of glioma malignancy that may affect therapeutic choices and patient outcome.[49] It has been reported that the correlation between the DCE-MR imaging metric $K^{trans}$ and tumor grade is weak and that rCBV is a more significant predictor of high-grade glioma than $K^{trans}$.[50]

Similar to DWI, signal-to-noise characteristics of (echo-planar imaging-based) perfusion MR imaging sequences are rather poor and voxel sizes tend to be large, as a result of which it may be difficult to exactly assess the extent of tumor spread in gliomas.[4]

Perfusion MR imaging techniques can depict changes in the internal architecture in the setting of no overall change in tumor size. For instance, because rCBV is thought to correspond to micro-vessel density, early response to antiangiogenesis therapy might manifest as a decrease in rCBV. Alternatively, because some angiogenesis factors are permeability promoters, a decreased rate of contrast material leakage (frequently quantified by means of $K^{trans}$) might be an early indication of response to antiangiogenesis therapy.[4] One study investigated the use of a voxel-based quantitative DSC-MR imaging approach (PRM of DSC-MR imaging metrics) for distinguishing pseudoprogression from true progression in patients with high-grade glioma.[51] The investigators of this study reported that 3 weeks after the start of concurrent chemoradiation therapy, a significantly increased PRM rCBV was noted in patients with progressive disease as compared with those with pseudoprogression. In contrast, change in average percent rCBV or rCBF, MR imaging tumor volume changes, age, extent of resection, and Radiation Therapy Oncology Group recursive partitioning analysis classification did not distinguish progression from pseudoprogression. Thus, a voxel-based analysis of rCBV at week 3 during chemoradiation therapy is a potential early imaging biomarker of response that may be helpful in distinguishing pseudoprogression from true progression in patients with high-grade glioma.[51] In another study, the same research group investigated the value of voxel-based analyses of changes in ADC (PRM$_{ADC}$) and

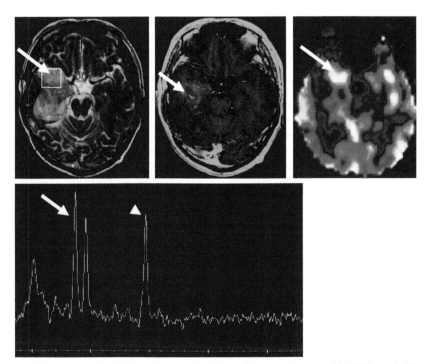

**Fig. 3.** Standard MR imaging, DSC-MR imaging, and MRS in a 64-year-old man with WHO grade III anaplastic oligodendroglioma. (*Top left*) The T2-weighted image shows a homogeneous mass in the right temporal lobe (*arrow*). The overlaid square indicates the position of the voxel for MRS. (*Top middle*) Inhomogeneous enhancement is demonstrated in the lesion (*arrow*). (*Top right*) The corresponding rCBV map clearly demonstrates areas of high vascularity (*arrow*). (*Bottom*) MRS data of the corresponding region demonstrate slightly increased choline (*arrow*) and relatively decreased NAA peaks (*arrowhead*), while no lactate peak is detected. (*Reproduced from* Toyooka M, Kimura H, Uematsu H, et al. Tissue characterization of glioma by proton magnetic resonance spectroscopy and perfusion-weighted magnetic resonance imaging: glioma grading and histologic correlation. Clin Imaging 2008;32(4):251–8; with permission.)

rCBV (PRMrCBV) in patients with high-grade glioma who received concurrent chemoradiation in predicting patient survival.[52] Their analysis showed that $PRM_{ADC}$ in combination with PRMrCBV obtained at week 3 had a stronger correlation to 1-year and overall survival rates than any baseline clinical or treatment response imaging metric. It was concluded that inclusion of $PRM_{ADC}$ and PRMrCBV into a single imaging biomarker metric allowed early identification of patients resistant to standard chemoradiation. In addition, in comparison to the current standard of assessment of response at 10 weeks (McDonald criteria), the composite PRM biomarker potentially provides a useful opportunity for clinicians to identify patients who may benefit from alternative treatment strategies.[52]

Based on the fact that high-grade gliomas are characterized by vascular proliferation,[2,3] the utility of perfusion MR imaging for discriminating tumor recurrence from radiation injury has been investigated by several studies.[28,53–55] These studies showed that the rCBV in recurrent high-grade glioma is significantly higher than in radiation necrosis.[28,53–55] Different studies have proposed different cutoff rCBV values for differentiating the 2 entities.[28,53–55] One prospective study demonstrated that a threshold value of 0.71 optimized differentiation of the histopathologic groups with a sensitivity of 91.7% and a specificity of 100%.[53] Regardless of the threshold value that is used, these data show that rCBV measurements may be able to differentiate high-grade glioma recurrence from posttreatment radiation effects with a high degree of accuracy.[28,53–55]

## MR SPECTROSCOPY
### Basic Principles

MRS is a molecular imaging method that allows for separation of the MR signal from a given tissue into its different chemical components, based on the principle of chemical shift.[56,57] MRS enables quantitative assessment of the amount, type, and location of small molecular compounds within a tissue or organ of interest. The data are typically displayed as a grid of spectra of chemical compound abundances obtained at either single or multiple locations in a tissue or organ of interest. Tissue volumes of less than 1 mL and metabolite concentrations less than 1 mM can be detected. In theory, MRS can be performed on any nucleus that exhibits nuclear spin. However, most substances are present in low quantities and are difficult to detect with conventional clinical systems. Proton ($^1$H) spectroscopy and phosphorus ($^{31}$P) spectroscopy, however, are feasible on most clinical systems, with phosphorous spectroscopy being largely limited to research applications investigating tissue energy production. The most frequently investigated metabolites in the proton spectrum include choline (Cho), N-acetylaspartate (NAA), lactate (Lac), lipid (Lip), and creatine (Cr). Cho is abundant in cell membranes, and the intensity of the Cho signal reflects changes in cell membrane synthesis and turnover. NAA is a neuronal marker, and the NAA signal is assumed to correspond to neuronal integrity. Lac is a product of anaerobic metabolism, and the intensity of the Lac signal may reflect ischemia and/or hypoxia. The presence of Lip peaks (provided that subcutaneous Lip has been suppressed well) is thought to be a result of necrosis. Finally, Cr includes both Cr and phosphocreatine, and the intensity of the Cr signal is often used as a reference to normalize the intensity of other metabolites.[56,57]

## Clinical Applications

Several studies have investigated the value of MRS for gliomas grading. For example, one study reported that grade III tumors had significantly higher Cho levels and average Cho/total NAA ratios than grade II tumors.[58] Another study reported that both maximum and mean Cho levels of high-grade gliomas are significantly higher than those of low-grade gliomas.[59] In addition, compared with contrast enhancement, mean Cho, and Cho/Cr, maximum Cho of the tumor provided the highest accuracy in discriminating between low- and high-grade tumors.[59] Despite the tendency of high-grade gliomas to have higher Cho levels, low-grade gliomas may also have elevated Cho levels, and Cho level peaks in grade IV tumors may be lower or equal to those in grade III tumors (the latter possibly due to micronecrosis in grade IV tumors).[48,60] Therefore, it remains questionable whether any of the Cho indices or ratios alone allow histologic grading of gliomas with sufficient diagnostic precision. Other (additional) metabolic markers such as Lac and Lip (which are typically elevated in high-grade

gliomas) may improve diagnostic accuracy and determination of prognosis.[61–63]

Multiple studies have shown that (high-grade) gliomas have elevated levels of Cho and decreased levels of NAA and Cr relative to normal brain tissue (see **Fig. 3**)[64–66] and that the changes in these metabolites are more sensitive than conventional contrast-enhanced MR imaging for the detection of tumor infiltration. Studies comparing MRS with tumor pathology have shown a correlation between the Cho peak and tumor cell density.[60,67] In addition, one study reported that in patients suspected of having glioma, biopsy samples containing tumor tissue could be distinguished from those containing a mixture of normal, edematous, gliotic, and necrotic tissue with 90% sensitivity and 86% specificity by using a cutoff Cho/NAA ratio of 2.5.[68] Of interest, about one-third to half of the T2-hyperintense lesion outside the contrast-enhancing lesion had a Cho/NAA ratio greater than 2.5.[68] Several studies have shown that patients with greater volumetric overlap between the radiosurgery target volume and the pretreatment metabolic abnormality (high Cho) volume tend to have better survival.[69,70] Another study reported a strong negative linear correlation between total NAA levels and both percentage of tumor infiltration and tumor cell number in biopsies from the border zone of gliomas but no correlation with Cho.[71] The researchers of this study postulated that these findings may be in accordance with the infiltrative nature of gliomas, leading to a displacement or destruction of neurons and therefore to a reduction in total NAA levels; this mechanism seems to take place in areas with low tumor infiltration. On the other hand, the increased anabolism of malignant cells in neoplastic lesions, which leads to rapid cell membrane proliferation and thus to increased Cho levels, occurs significantly only at higher tumor cell infiltration.[71] One should be aware that treatment and inflammation may result in metabolic changes in non–tumor-infiltrated brain tissue; a transient increase in Cho levels and a decrease in NAA levels have been reported in the first 4 to 6 months after radiation therapy.[72,73]

The value of MRS in early response assessment has not been established yet. A reduction in Cho level within the tumor has been demonstrated to parallel a decrease in tumor volume during chemotherapy.[74–76] Although some studies have suggested spectral changes (in particular Cho-containing compounds) over the course of time to be predictive of therapeutic response (**Fig. 4**),[77–80] other studies were not able to demonstrate a prognostic value of MRS parameters.[81] Limitations of these initial studies are their limited

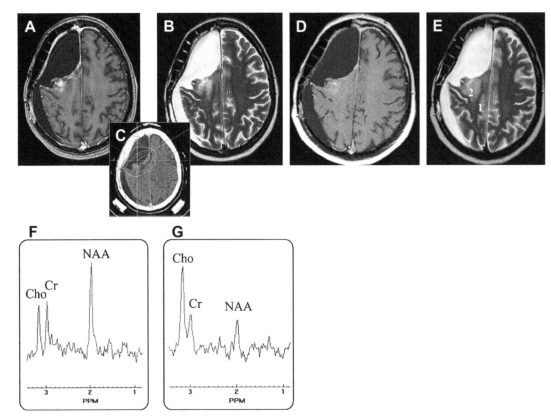

**Fig. 4.** A 48-year-old patient with anaplastic oligodendroglioma, initially WHO grade II. Two years after primary surgery, reoperation combined with external-beam irradiation (56 Gy) was performed. Two years later, further tumor progression was observed, and after excision, a procarbazine, lomustine, and vincristine-chemotherapy was applied. After completion of 9 months of the last cycle of chemotherapy, further growth and new contrast enhancement were obvious (*A, B*). Fractionated stereotactic boost radiation therapy (36 Gy) was therefore conducted (*C*). The first follow-up showed a reduction in contrast enhancing 4 months later (*D*), whereas slight growth of T2-hyperintense area and elevation of Cho levels [reference spectrum localization (1) is given in (*E*) and shown in (*F*), spectra 2 within suspicious lesion is given in (*G*)] revealed failure of local tumor control. Clinical symptoms aggravated, and 5 months later, the patient was hospitalized because of multifocal recurrence with subependyma sowings. (*Reproduced from* Lichy MP, Plathow C, Schulz-Ertner D, et al. Follow-up gliomas after radiotherapy: 1H MR spectroscopic imaging for increasing diagnostic accuracy. Neuroradiology 2005;47(11):826–34; with permission.)

sample sizes, necessitating further research in larger patient populations.

MRS may be a valuable method to discriminate radiation injury from glioma recurrence. Dose-dependent, specific metabolic changes have been reported to occur after radiation therapy, including a decrease in NAA levels and variable changes in Cho and Cr levels.[72,73,82] Unfortunately, in many of the new enhancing regions, both tumor cells and radiation injury are present, and the spectral patterns in such cases are less definitive than in pure tumor or radiation necrosis.[27,82] Nevertheless, several metabolic ratios such as Cho/NAA and Cho/Cr have been repeatedly reported to be significantly higher in recurrent tumor than in radiation injury, and investigators have shown that these allow discrimination of the 2 entities with moderate to good diagnostic precision.[27,83–86] For example, in a 2011 study, Cho/NAA and NAA/Cr ratios have been reported to provide sensitivities and specificities for the prediction of tumor recurrence of 86% and 90%, and 93% and 70%, respectively.[86]

## PET/MR IMAGING
### Basic Principles

The first decade of the twenty-first century has seen a steep increase in the clinical usage of combined (or hybrid) PET/computed tomographic (CT) scanners. The advantages of combining functional and anatomic information are more than just the sum of the advantages of the separate modalities.[87,88] Ten years after the first clinical PET/CT scanner, another combined imaging technology appeared: the combined PET/MR imaging. So, will the PET/MR imaging follow in the footsteps of or even supersede the PET/CT? Using MR imaging instead of CT in conjunction with PET has some major advantages. First, MR imaging provides far better soft-tissue contrast compared with CT. Second, MR imaging does not impose additional radiation unlike CT.[88] In addition, MR imaging offers the ability to provide functional information as described earlier. Hence, PET/MR imaging holds promise of being the ideal multimodality imaging technology.

Several PET/MR imaging system layouts have been developed and tested. Unlike PET/CT, combined PET/MR imaging cannot be realized by just coupling 2 existing technologies. The components of the PET and MR imaging systems can easily influence each other, which leads to severe image degradation of either modality. Three vendors have introduced clinical PET/MR imaging systems, all with a different approach.[89] One approach is to separate the PET and MR image components and transfer the immobilized patient from PET to MR imaging. This way, interference between the PET and MR imaging systems is minimized. Major drawbacks are that images are acquired sequentially and not simultaneously, inducing a potentially unwanted temporal factor between PET and MR imaging data, leading to long acquisition times and (still) the possibility of misalignment due to patient movement. A fully integrated PET/MR imaging system has the highest potential but is at the same time technically the most challenging (**Fig. 5**). To be able to acquire PET and MR images simultaneously, several technological hurdles have to be overcome.

One of the major problems is the magnetic susceptibility of the photomultiplier tube (PMT), which is a crucial component of PET systems. Gamma photons emitted from the patient are converted into weak light pulses in the PET detectors' crystal, which in turn are converted into small electrical pulses that are processed by the computer system to build up an image.[90] Because PMTs basically consist of vacuum tubes using a high electric field to accelerate electrons, they are easily influenced by even weak external magnetic fields. Furthermore, they are bulky and would narrow the ring bore too much when fitted in a standard MR imaging ring.

Alternatives have been developed, such as fiberoptics, to carry the scintillation signal to a shielded PMT outside the MR imaging fringe field and semiconductor detectors.[90] The avalanche photodiode and silicon photomultiplier have shown promising results and have even been used in some clinical PET/MR imaging systems.

Owing to their compact size and their insensitivity even to high magnetic fields they are used instead of conventional PMTs in a combined PET/MR imaging system.[90,91]

PET components can also influence the MR image quality. Potential interfering factors that have to be taken into account are the magnetic susceptibility, the conductivity, and the electric resistance of the PET components, leading to specific requirements for, among other PET components, the scintillation crystal and the gamma shielding material, which is needed to minimize random events in the PET system.[91,92]

Another complicating factor is PET attenuation correction, which is needed to correct for the tissue attenuation of the annihilation gamma photons. Using an external radiation source to create a transmission map like in the older stand-alone PET systems is unfavorable because of the additional radiation, time consumption, and space requirements. In PET/CT systems, the CT image, reflecting the electron density, is used directly as an attenuation map. The MR imaging data, however, reflect the proton density, which is not directly related to gamma photon attenuation. Specific MR imaging sequences and MR imaging data processing are needed to use MR imaging as attenuation correction.[90,93]

### Clinical Applications

Neuroimaging has always been an important share of PET and MR imaging, and both imaging modalities have proved their value in glioma imaging.[94] However, despite technological feasibility, do we need combined PET/MR imaging in glioma imaging?

Although simultaneous acquisition allows for perfect coregistration, software fusion of separate PET and MR imaging data in brain imaging is easy compared with less rigid body structures and has proved to have added clinical value (**Fig. 6**).[94,95] However, combined PET/MR imaging has several advantages over separate PET and MR imaging. Combined PET/MR imaging can provide simultaneous information from MR imaging (morphology, DWI, perfusion, DTI, and MRS) and PET (eg, blood flow, glucose metabolism, oxygen consumption, and amino acid and nucleoside uptake).[96] It is possible to correlate MR imaging and PET data real time, providing even more insight into the relationship between PET and MR imaging parameters and facilitating cross-validation of the 2 modalities. Furthermore, PET/MR imaging might be used when timely imaging from both modalities is needed. For instance, in clinical neurosciences, PET combined with DTI might reveal the relationship between transmitter release, receptor

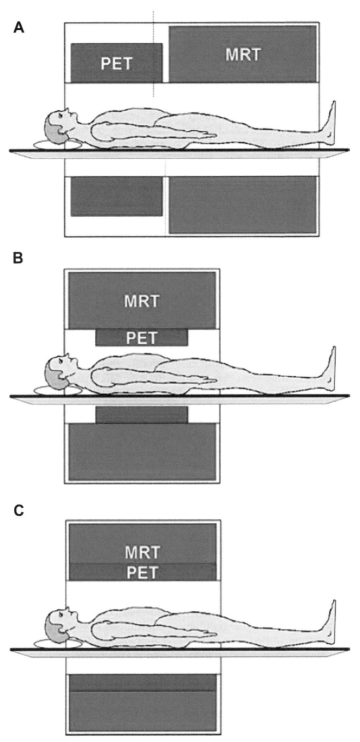

Fig. 5. Several PET/MR imaging system layouts. PET/MR imaging system with back-to-back layout (like PET/CT) allowing sequential, although not simultaneous, imaging (*A*); standard MR imaging system, with MR imaging-compatible PET insert, reducing system costs but creating space constraints (*B*); fully integrated PET/MR imaging system allowing versatile application of simultaneous PET/MR imaging (*C*). (*Reproduced from* Pichler BJ, Judenhofer MS, Wehrl HF. PET/MRI hybrid imaging: devices and initial results. Eur Radiol 2008;18(3):1077–86, with permission.)

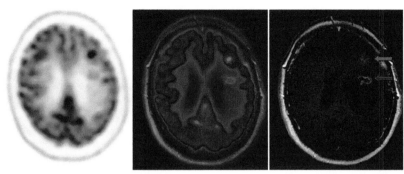

Fig. 6. A 68-year-old patient with recurrent glioblastoma multiforme (WHO grade IV). Eleven months after resection and combined chemoradiation therapy, a new, contrast-enhancing lesion (*red arrow*) was seen on a follow-up T1-weighted MR image in the left frontal lobe (*right*), which was not seen on an MR scan 6 weeks earlier (not shown). To confirm recurrence of malignancy and to exclude radiation necrosis, 4 days later [18]F-FDG-PET/CT was performed ([18]F-FDG-PET combined with low-dose CT; CT not shown), showing a hypermetabolic left frontal lobe lesion (*left*). Semiautomated fusion using syngo.via imaging software (Siemens Healthcare, Forchheim, Germany) shows perfect match of the [18]F-FDG-PET hypermetabolic focus and the new, contrast-enhancing lesion on MR imaging (*middle*), consistent with tumor recurrence. The rim-enhancing resection cavity on T1-weighted MR imaging (*blue arrow*), which had been stable on multiple MR scans during the 11 months of follow-up, shows just minimal [18]F-FDG uptake, indicating the absence of (macroscopic) malignancy at this location.

occupancy, and functional neuronal networks during or just after cognitive tasks. In addition, when work processes are streamlined, combined PET/MR imaging might prove to be more time efficient than separate imaging.

The first combined PET/MR imaging study in humans was a combined [18]F-FDG-PET/MR brain imaging study performed in 2006 on 2 patients just after a PET/CT for other clinical reasons.[97] No obvious interference between PET and MR image quality was observed, showing the feasibility of combined clinical PET/MR imaging.

So far, there is only one clinical study that used combined PET/MR imaging for the evaluation of brain tumors.[98] In this small study (n = 10), 6 patients with (suspicion of) glioma were included, among patients with other primary brain tumors. These 6 patients underwent [11]C-methionine PET combined with standard morphologic MR imaging sequences, just after a clinically indicated PET/CT. The investigators found comparable PET image quality between the PET/MR imaging and PET/CT studies and no noticeable artifacts on the magnetic resonance images. Moreover, there was an excellent tumor-to-reference tissue ratio accordance between the PET images performed on the different modalities. However, when scanning in high-resolution mode, streak artifacts were visible on PET images in the sagittal and coronal directions, likely due to the large gaps between the PET detector blocks.

Recent developments have shown that clinical combined PET/MR imaging is technically feasible but far from consolidated.

As the combined PET/MR imaging is at the doorstep of more widespread clinical application, further studies are needed to optimize scanning parameters and work processes and to prove added value and cost-effectiveness.

## SUMMARY

A selection of important advanced MR imaging techniques (DWI, DTI, perfusion MR imaging, and MRS) and the evolving role of PET/MR imaging in the evaluation of high-grade gliomas in various settings have been reviewed in this article. It is important to consider these potentially useful imaging methods as complementary; a multiparametric approach is expected to provide better evaluation of high-grade gliomas (and brain tumors in general) than either of the methods alone. Future research should (1) technically optimize these advanced imaging methods and determine their reproducibility to enable more widespread implementation, (2) more rigorously investigate which (combination) of these advanced imaging methods provides superior diagnostic and prognostic information compared with current standard imaging methods, (3) determine whether these advanced imaging methods improve patient survival and are cost-effective.

## REFERENCES

1. Siegel R, Naishadham D, Jemal A. Cancer statistics, 2012. CA Cancer J Clin 2012;62(1):10–29.

2. Behin A, Hoang-Xuan K, Carpentier AF, et al. Primary brain tumours in adults. Lancet 2003; 361(9354):323–31.

3. Reardon DA, Rich JN, Friedman HS, et al. Recent advances in the treatment of malignant astrocytoma. J Clin Oncol 2006;24(8):1253–65.

4. Provenzale JM, Mukundan S, Barboriak DP. Diffusion-weighted and perfusion MR imaging for brain tumor characterization and assessment of treatment response. Radiology 2006;239(3):632–49.

5. Einstein A. Investigations on the theory of the Brownian motion. New York: Dover; 1956.

6. Bammer R. Basic principles of diffusion-weighted imaging. Eur J Radiol 2003;45(3):169–84.

7. Sotak CH. Nuclear magnetic resonance (NMR) measurement of the apparent diffusion coefficient (ADC) of tissue water and its relationship to cell volume changes in pathological states. Neurochem Int 2004;45(4):569–82.

8. Stejskal EO, Tanner JE. Spin diffusion measurements: spin echoes in the presence of a time-dependent field gradient. J Chem Phys 1965; 42(1):288–92.

9. De Figueiredo EH, Borgonovi AF, Doring TM. Basic concepts of MR imaging, diffusion MR imaging, and diffusion tensor imaging. Magn Reson Imaging Clin N Am 2011;19(1):1–22.

10. Le Bihan D. Molecular diffusion nuclear magnetic resonance imaging. Magn Reson Q 1991;7(1):1–30.

11. Murakami R, Hirai T, Sugahara T, et al. Grading astrocytic tumors by using apparent diffusion coefficient parameters: superiority of a one- versus two-parameter pilot method. Radiology 2009;251(3): 838–45.

12. Kang Y, Choi SH, Kim YJ, et al. Gliomas: histogram analysis of apparent diffusion coefficient maps with standard- or high-b-value diffusion-weighted MR imaging–correlation with tumor grade. Radiology 2011;261(3):882–90.

13. Johnson PC, Hunt SJ, Drayer BP. Human cerebral gliomas: correlation of postmortem imaging findings and neuropathologic findings. Radiology 1989; 170(1 Pt 1):211–7.

14. Oh J, Henry RG, Pirzkall A, et al. Survival analysis in patients with glioblastoma multiforme: predictive value of choline-to-N-acetylaspartate index, apparent diffusion coefficient, and relative cerebral blood volume. J Magn Reson Imaging 2004;19(5):546–54.

15. Pauleit D, Langen KJ, Floeth F, et al. Can the apparent diffusion coefficient be used as a noninvasive parameter to distinguish tumor tissue from peritumoral tissue in cerebral gliomas? J Magn Reson Imaging 2004;20(5):758–64.

16. Macdonald DR, Cascino TL, Schold SC Jr, et al. Response criteria for phase II studies of supratentorial malignant glioma. J Clin Oncol 1990;8(7): 1277–80.

17. Brandsma D, van den Bent MJ. Pseudoprogression and pseudoresponse in the treatment of gliomas. Curr Opin Neurol 2009;22(6):633–8.

18. Wen PY, Macdonald DR, Reardon DA, et al. Updated response assessment criteria for high-grade gliomas: response assessment in neuro-oncology working group. J Clin Oncol 2010; 28(11):1963–72.

19. Hamstra DA, Rehemtulla A, Ross BD. Diffusion magnetic resonance imaging: a biomarker for treatment response in oncology. J Clin Oncol 2007; 25(26):4104–9.

20. Hamstra DA, Galbán CJ, Meyer CR, et al. Functional diffusion map as an early imaging biomarker for high-grade glioma: correlation with conventional radiologic response and overall survival. J Clin Oncol 2008;26(20):3387–94.

21. Ellingson BM, Malkin MG, Rand SD, et al. Volumetric analysis of functional diffusion maps is a predictive imaging biomarker for cytotoxic and anti-angiogenic treatments in malignant gliomas. J Neurooncol 2011;102(1):95–103.

22. Hygino da Cruz LC Jr, Rodriguez I, Domingues RC, et al. Pseudoprogression and pseudoresponse imaging challenges in the assessment of posttreatment glioma. AJNR Am J Neuroradiol 2011;32(11): 1978–85.

23. Padhani AR, Liu G, Koh DM, et al. Diffusion-weighted magnetic resonance imaging as a cancer biomarker: consensus and recommendations. Neoplasia 2009;11(2):102–25.

24. Hein PA, Eskey CJ, Dunn JF, et al. Diffusion-weighted imaging in the follow-up of treated high-grade gliomas: tumor recurrence versus radiation injury. AJNR Am J Neuroradiol 2004;25(2):201–9.

25. Sundgren PC, Fan X, Weybright P, et al. Differentiation of recurrent brain tumor versus radiation injury using diffusion tensor imaging in patients with new contrast-enhancing lesions. Magn Reson Imaging 2006;24(9):1131–42.

26. Xu JL, Li YL, Lian JM, et al. Distinction between postoperative recurrent glioma and radiation injury using MR diffusion tensor imaging. Neuroradiology 2010; 52(12):1193–9.

27. Rock JP, Scarpace L, Hearshen D, et al. Associations among magnetic resonance spectroscopy, apparent diffusion coefficients, and image-guided histopathology with special attention to radiation necrosis. Neurosurgery 2004;54(5):1111–7.

28. Bobek-Billewicz B, Stasik-Pres G, Majchrzak H, et al. Differentiation between brain tumor recurrence and radiation injury using perfusion, diffusion-weighted imaging and MR spectroscopy. Folia Neuropathol 2010;48(2):81–92.

29. Beaulieu C. The basis of anisotropic water diffusion in the nervous system - a technical review. NMR Biomed 2002;15(7–8):435–55.

30. Le Bihan D, Mangin JF, Poupon C, et al. Diffusion tensor imaging: concepts and applications. J Magn Reson Imaging 2001;13(4):534–46.

31. Berman J. Diffusion MR tractography as a tool for surgical planning. Magn Reson Imaging Clin N Am 2009;17(2):205–14.

32. Inoue T, Ogasawara K, Beppu T, et al. Diffusion tensor imaging for preoperative evaluation of tumor grade in gliomas. Clin Neurol Neurosurg 2005; 107(3):174–80.

33. Liu X, Tian W, Kolar B, et al. MR diffusion tensor and perfusion-weighted imaging in preoperative grading of supratentorial nonenhancing gliomas. Neuro Oncol 2011;13(4):447–55.

34. Lu S, Ahn D, Johnson G, et al. Diffusion-tensor MR imaging of intracranial neoplasia and associated peritumoral edema: introduction of the tumor infiltration index. Radiology 2004;232(1):221–8.

35. Lee HY, Na DG, Song IC, et al. Diffusion-tensor imaging for glioma grading at 3-T magnetic resonance imaging: analysis of fractional anisotropy and mean diffusivity. J Comput Assist Tomogr 2008;32(2):298–303.

36. Price SJ, Burnet NG, Donovan T, et al. Diffusion tensor imaging of brain tumours at 3T: a potential tool for assessing white matter tract invasion? Clin Radiol 2003;58(6):455–62.

37. Provenzale JM, McGraw P, Mhatre P, et al. Peritumoral brain regions in gliomas and meningiomas: investigation with isotropic diffusion-weighted MR imaging and diffusion-tensor MR imaging. Radiology 2004;232(2):451–60.

38. Stadlbauer A, Ganslandt O, Buslei R, et al. Gliomas: histopathologic evaluation of changes in directionality and magnitude of water diffusion at diffusion-tensor MR imaging. Radiology 2006;240(3):803–10.

39. Price SJ, Jena R, Burnet NG, et al. Improved delineation of glioma margins and regions of infiltration with the use of diffusion tensor imaging: an image-guided biopsy study. AJNR Am J Neuroradiol 2006;27(9):1969–74.

40. Price SJ, Jena R, Burnet NG, et al. Predicting patterns of glioma recurrence using diffusion tensor imaging. Eur Radiol 2007;17(7):1675–84.

41. Deprez S, Amant F, Smeets A, et al. Longitudinal assessment of chemotherapy-induced structural changes in cerebral white matter and its correlation with impaired cognitive functioning. J Clin Oncol 2012;30(3):274–81.

42. Lope-Piedrafita S, Garcia-Martin ML, Galons JP, et al. Longitudinal diffusion tensor imaging in a rat brain glioma model. NMR Biomed 2008;21(8):799–808.

43. Kashimura H, Inoue T, Beppu T, et al. Diffusion tensor imaging for differentiation of recurrent brain tumor and radiation necrosis after radiotherapy—three case reports. Clin Neurol Neurosurg 2007; 109(1):106–10.

44. Padhani AR. Dynamic contrast-enhanced MR imaging. Cancer Imaging 2000;1(1):52–63.

45. Hylton N. Dynamic contrast-enhanced magnetic resonance imaging as an imaging biomarker. J Clin Oncol 2006;24(20):3293–8.

46. Kwee TC, Takahara T, Klomp DW, et al. Cancer imaging: novel concepts in clinical magnetic resonance imaging. J Intern Med 2010;268(2):120–32.

47. Essig M, Anzalone N, Combs SE, et al. MR imaging of neoplastic central nervous system lesions: review and recommendations for current practice. AJNR Am J Neuroradiol 2012;33(5):803–17.

48. Law M, Yang S, Wang H, et al. Glioma grading: sensitivity, specificity, and predictive values of perfusion MR imaging and proton MR spectroscopic imaging compared with conventional MR imaging. AJNR Am J Neuroradiol 2003;24(10):1989–98.

49. Law M, Young RJ, Babb JS, et al. Gliomas: predicting time to progression or survival with cerebral blood volume measurements at dynamic susceptibility-weighted contrast-enhanced perfusion MR imaging. Radiology 2008;247(2):490–8.

50. Law M, Yang S, Babb JS, et al. Comparison of cerebral blood volume and vascular permeability from dynamic susceptibility contrast-enhanced perfusion MR imaging with glioma grade. AJNR Am J Neuroradiol 2004;25(5):746–55.

51. Tsien C, Galbán CJ, Chenevert TL, et al. Parametric response map as an imaging biomarker to distinguish progression from pseudoprogression in high-grade glioma. J Clin Oncol 2010;28(13): 2293–9.

52. Galbán CJ, Chenevert TL, Meyer CR, et al. Prospective analysis of parametric response map-derived MRI biomarkers: identification of early and distinct glioma response patterns not predicted by standard radiographic assessment. Clin Cancer Res 2011; 17(14):4751–60.

53. Hu LS, Baxter LC, Smith KA, et al. Relative cerebral blood volume values to differentiate high-grade glioma recurrence from posttreatment radiation effect: direct correlation between image-guided tissue histopathology and localized dynamic susceptibility-weighted contrast-enhanced perfusion MR imaging measurements. AJNR Am J Neuroradiol 2009;30(3):552–8.

54. Kim YH, Oh SW, Lim YJ, et al. Differentiating radiation necrosis from tumor recurrence in high-grade gliomas: assessing the efficacy of 18F-FDG PET, 11C-methionine PET and perfusion MRI. Clin Neurol Neurosurg 2010;112(9):758–65.

55. Xu JL, Shi DP, Dou SW, et al. Distinction between postoperative recurrent gliomas and delayed radiation injury using MR perfusion weighted imaging. J Med Imaging Radiat Oncol 2011;55(6):587–94.

56. Aisen AM, Chenevert TL. MR spectroscopy: clinical perspective. Radiology 1989;173(3):593–9.

57. Mountford C, Lean C, Malycha P, et al. Proton spectroscopy provides accurate pathology on biopsy and in vivo. J Magn Reson Imaging 2006;24(3): 459–77.

58. Stadlbauer A, Gruber S, Nimsky C, et al. Preoperative grading of gliomas by using metabolite quantification with high-spatial-resolution proton MR spectroscopic imaging. Radiology 2006;283(3): 958–69.

59. Senft C, Hattingen E, Pilatus U, et al. Diagnostic value of proton magnetic resonance spectroscopy in the noninvasive grading of solid gliomas: comparison of maximum and mean choline values. Neurosurgery 2009;65(5):908–13.

60. Croteau D, Scarpace L, Hearshen D, et al. Correlation between magnetic resonance spectroscopy imaging and image-guided biopsies: semiquantitative and qualitative histopathological analysis of patients with untreated gliomas. Neurosurgery 2001;49(4):823–9.

61. Fayed N, Morales H, Modrego PJ, et al. Contrast/noise ratio on conventional MRI and choline/creatine ratio on proton MRI spectroscopy accurately discriminate low-grade from high-grade cerebral gliomas. Acad Radiol 2006;13(6):728–37.

62. Toyooka M, Kimura H, Uematsu H, et al. Tissue characterization of glioma by proton magnetic resonance spectroscopy and perfusion-weighted magnetic resonance imaging: glioma grading and histological correlation. Clin Imaging 2008;32(4): 251–8.

63. Crawford FW, Khayal IS, McGue C, et al. Relationship of pre-surgery metabolic and physiological imaging parameters to survival for patients with untreated GBM. J Neurooncol 2009;91(3):337–51.

64. Cheng LL, Chang IW, Louis DN, et al. Correlation of high-resolution magic angle spinning proton magnetic resonance spectroscopy with histopathology of intact human brain tumor specimens. Cancer Res 1998;58(9):1825–32.

65. Kinoshita Y, Yokota A. Absolute concentrations of metabolites in human brain tumors using in vitro proton magnetic resonance spectroscopy. NMR Biomed 1997;10(1):2–12.

66. Poptani H, Gupta RK, Roy R, et al. Characterization of intracranial mass lesions with in vivo proton MR spectroscopy. AJNR Am J Neuroradiol 1995;16(8): 1593–603.

67. Nafe R, Herminghaus S, Raab P, et al. Preoperative proton-MR spectroscopy of gliomas–correlation with quantitative nuclear morphology in surgical specimen. J Neurooncol 2003;63(3):233–45.

68. McKnight TR, Von dem Bussche MH, Vigneron DB, et al. Histopathological validation of a three-dimensional magnetic resonance spectroscopy index as a predictor of tumor presence. J Neurosurg 2002;97(4):794–802.

69. Graves EE, Nelson SJ, Vigneron DB, et al. A preliminary study of the prognostic value of proton magnetic resonance spectroscopic imaging in gamma knife radiosurgery of recurrent malignant gliomas. Neurosurgery 2000;46(2):319–26.

70. Chan AA, Lau A, Pirzkall A, et al. Proton magnetic resonance spectroscopy imaging in the evaluation of patients undergoing gamma knife surgery for grade IV glioma. J Neurosurg 2004;101(3):467–75.

71. Stadlbauer A, Nimsky C, Buslei R, et al. Proton magnetic resonance spectroscopy in the border zone of gliomas: correlation of metabolic and histologic changes at low tumor infiltration – initial results. Invest Radiol 2007;42(4):218–23.

72. Esteve F, Rubin C, Grand S, et al. Transient metabolic changes in normal human brain after radiation therapy. Int J Radiat Oncol Biol Phys 1998;40(2): 279–86.

73. Lee MC, Pirzkall A, McKnight TR, et al. 1H-MRSI of radiation effects in normal-appearing white matter: dose dependence and impact on automated spectral classification. J Magn Reson Imaging 2004; 19(4):379–88.

74. Weber MA, Giesel FL, Stieltjes B. MRI for identification of progression in brain tumors: from morphology to function. Expert Rev Neurother 2008;8(10):1507–25.

75. Murphy PS, Viviers L, Abson C, et al. Monitoring temozolomide treatment of low-grade glioma with proton magnetic resonance spectroscopy. Br J Cancer 2004;90(4):781–6.

76. Lichy MP, Plathow C, Schulz-Ertner D, et al. Follow-up gliomas after radiotherapy: 1H MR spectroscopic imaging for increasing diagnostic accuracy. Neuroradiology 2005;47(11):826–34.

77. Preul MC, Caramanos Z, Villemure JG, et al. Using proton magnetic resonance spectroscopic imaging to predict in vivo the response of recurrent malignant gliomas to tamoxifen chemotherapy. Neurosurgery 2000;46(2):306–18.

78. Alexander A, Murtha A, Abdulkarim B, et al. Prognostic significance of serial magnetic resonance spectroscopies over the course of radiation therapy for patients with malignant glioma. Clin Invest Med 2006;29(5):301–11.

79. Guillevin R, Menuel C, Taillibert S, et al. Predicting the outcome of grade II glioma treated with temozolomide using proton magnetic resonance spectroscopy. Br J Cancer 2011;104(12):1854–61.

80. Quon H, Brunet B, Alexander A, et al. Changes in serial magnetic resonance spectroscopy predict outcome in high-grade glioma during and after postoperative radiotherapy. Anticancer Res 2011;31(10): 3559–65.

81. Vöglein J, Tüttenberg J, Weimer M, et al. Treatment monitoring in gliomas: comparison of dynamic susceptibility-weighted contrast-enhanced and

spectroscopic MRI techniques for identifying treatment failure. Invest Radiol 2011;46(6):390–400.

82. Cao Y, Sundgren PC, Tsien CI, et al. Physiologic and metabolic magnetic resonance imaging in gliomas. J Clin Oncol 2006;24(8):1228–35.

83. Weybright P, Sundgren PC, Maly P, et al. Differentiation between brain tumor recurrence and radiation injury using MR spectroscopy. AJR Am J Roentgenol 2005;185(6):1471–6.

84. Zeng QS, Li CF, Zhang K, et al. Multivoxel 3D proton MR spectroscopy in the distinction of recurrent glioma from radiation injury. J Neurooncol 2007; 84(1):63–9.

85. Smith EA, Carlos RC, Junck LR, et al. Developing a clinical decision model: MR spectroscopy to differentiate between recurrent tumor and radiation change in patients with new contrast-enhancing lesions. AJR Am J Roentgenol 2009;192(2):W45–52.

86. Elias AE, Carlos RC, Smith EA, et al. MR spectroscopy using normalized and non-normalized metabolite ratios for differentiating recurrent brain tumor from radiation injury. Acad Radiol 2011;18(9):1101–8.

87. Hany TF, Steinert HC, Goerres GW, et al. PET diagnostic accuracy: improvement with in-line PET-CT system: initial results. Radiology 2002; 225(2):575–81.

88. Hicks R, Lau E, Binns D. Hybrid imaging is the future of molecular imaging. Biomed Imaging Interv J 2007;3(3):e49.

89. Beyer T, Freudenberg LS, Czernin J, et al. The future of hybrid imaging - part 3: PET/MR, small-animal imaging and beyond. Insights Imaging 2011;2: 235–46.

90. Pichler BJ, Judenhofer MS, Wehrl HF. PET/MRI hybrid imaging: devices and initial results. Eur Radiol 2008;18(3):1077–86.

91. Lecomte R. Novel detector technology for clinical PET. Eur J Nucl Med Mol Imaging 2009; 36(Suppl 1):S69–85.

92. Yamamoto S, Watabe T, Watabe H, et al. Simultaneous imaging using Si-PM-based PET and MRI for development of an integrated PET/MRI system. Phys Med Biol 2012;57(2):N1–13.

93. Berker Y, Franke J, Salomon A, et al. MRI-based attenuation correction for hybrid PET/MRI systems: a 4-class tissue segmentation technique using a combined ultrashort-echo-time/Dixon MRI sequence. J Nucl Med 2012;53(5):796–804.

94. Chen W. Clinical applications of PET in brain tumors. J Nucl Med 2007;48(9):1468–81.

95. Borgwardt L, Højgaard L, Carstensen H, et al. Increased fluorine-18 2-fluoro-2-deoxy-D-glucose (FDG) uptake in childhood CNS tumors is correlated with malignancy grade: a study with FDG positron emission tomography/magnetic resonance imaging coregistration and image fusion. J Clin Oncol 2005;23(13):3030–7.

96. Heiss WD. The potential of PET/MR for brain imaging. Eur J Nucl Med Mol Imaging 2009; 36(Suppl 1):S105–12.

97. Schlemmer HP, Pichler BJ, Schmand M, et al. Simultaneous MR/PET imaging of the human brain: feasibility study. Radiology 2008;248(3):1028–35.

98. Boss A, Bisdas S, Kolb A, et al. Hybrid PET/MRI of intracranial masses: initial experiences and comparison to PET/CT. J Nucl Med 2010;51(8):1198–205.

# PET Parametric Response Mapping for Clinical Monitoring and Treatment Response Evaluation in Brain Tumors

Benjamin M. Ellingson, PhD[a,b,c,*], Wei Chen, MD[d],
Robert J. Harris, BS[a,b], Whitney B. Pope, MD, PhD[a],
Albert Lai, MD, PhD[e], Phioanh L. Nghiemphu, MD[e],
Johannes Czernin, MD[d], Michael E. Phelps, PhD[d],
Timothy F. Cloughesy, MD[e]

## KEYWORDS

- PET • PET parametric response maps • Glioblastoma • GBM • Brain tumors • Imaging • Response
- Biomarker

## KEY POINTS

- PET parametric response maps (PRMs) are a personalized imaging biomarker for quantifying regional changes in PET tracer uptake over time.
- PET PRMs evaluated from PET images before and after therapy can be used to visualize and quantify heterogeneous brain tumor response and predict survival.
- Response to therapy using PET PRMs can vary depending on the PET tracer used for evaluation.
- PET PRMs evaluated over time can be used to monitor tumor growth, particularly in slow-growing low-grade brain tumors.

## INTRODUCTION

Gliomas account for more than 30% of all primary brain and central nervous system tumors, making up more than 80% of all malignant brain tumors.[1]

Malignant gliomas are the second leading cause of cancer mortality in people younger than age 35, the fourth leading cause in those younger than age 54, and kill approximately 13,000 people per year.[1] Glioblastoma is one of the most

Funding: UCLA Institute for Molecular Medicine Seed Grant (BME); UCLA Radiology Exploratory Research Grant (BME); University of California Cancer Research Coordinating Committee Grant (BME); ACRIN Young Investigator Initiative Grant (BME); Art of the Brain (TFC); Ziering Family Foundation in memory of Sigi Ziering (TFC); Singleton Family Foundation (TFC); Clarence Klein Fund for Neuro-Oncology (TFC).
[a] Department of Radiological Sciences, David Geffen School of Medicine, University of California Los Angeles, Los Angeles, CA, USA; [b] Department of Biomedical Physics, David Geffen School of Medicine, University of California Los Angeles, Los Angeles, CA, USA; [c] Department of Biomedical Engineering, David Geffen School of Medicine, University of California Los Angeles, Los Angeles, CA, USA; [d] Department of Molecular and Medical Pharmacology, David Geffen School of Medicine, University of California Los Angeles, Los Angeles, CA, USA; [e] Department of Neurology, David Geffen School of Medicine, University of California Los Angeles, Los Angeles, CA, USA
* Corresponding author. Department of Radiological Sciences, David Geffen School of Medicine, University of California Los Angeles, 924 Westwood Boulevard, Suite 615, Los Angeles, CA 90024.
*E-mail address:* bellingson@mednet.ucla.edu

PET Clin 8 (2013) 201–217
http://dx.doi.org/10.1016/j.cpet.2012.09.002
1556-8598/13/$ – see front matter © 2013 Elsevier Inc. All rights reserved.

aggressive types of malignant brain tumors, having only a mean survival of around 14.6 months with standard radiation and chemotherapy,[2] which has not changed appreciably in the last 50 years. This dismal prognosis is attributed to many factors; however, the use of relatively ineffective single-agent treatments for genetic heterogeneous tumors, along with tumor growth and invasion not detected with current imaging techniques, are the major barriers for improving survival.

Although ineffective treatments and limitations in standard imaging techniques may seem to be mutually exclusive issues, they are in fact intertwined. The effectiveness of treatments is largely determined by tumor progression defined by imaging. Serial imaging of brain tumors over time is currently the best way of monitoring a patient's progress on different treatments and currently is the most accepted method of quantifying brain tumor progression. T1-weighted MR imaging with the use of gadolinium contrast agents is the most robust and widely used method of determining treatment failure[3]; however, with the recent advent of antiangiogenic therapies in brain tumors this may no longer be the case. Antiangiogenic drugs that target tumor vasculature are known to reduce vascular permeability, resulting in a decrease in contrast enhancement on postcontrast T1-weighted MR images, independent of potential antitumor effects. Additionally, many brain tumors (particular low-grade tumors) do not present with contrast enhancement, thus this type of imaging is of limited use. For this reason, the Response Assessment in Neuro-Oncology working group was established and has proposed new guidelines for determining brain tumor progression,[4] including the use of T2-weighted or fluid-attenuated inversion recovery images to help delineate permeability changes from nonenhancing tumor spread. These real-world challenges associated with detecting tumor growth, invasion, and treatment response using conventional MR imaging in the current era of clinical neuro-oncology treatment provide the unique opportunity for molecular imaging techniques, including PET, to play a pivotal role in the management of patients with brain tumors.

## COMMON PET TRACERS IN BRAIN TUMORS

PET radiotracers have been used for the evaluation of brain tumors as early as 1982, when Di Chiro and colleagues[5] synthesized and used [$^{18}$F]-fluorodeoxyglucose ($^{18}$F-FDG) to characterize hypermetabolism in brain tumors. In follow-up studies, Di Chiro[6] clearly demonstrated the ability for $^{18}$F-

FDG uptake to predict patient survival, even better than histologic grading. Since these early studies, $^{18}$F-FDG has been used in a great many studies[7] for determining initial diagnosis,[8,9] identifying tumor recurrence,[10–14] grading of brain tumors,[15,16] identification of treatment response to radiotherapy,[17] cytotoxic therapeutics,[18,19] and antiangiogenic therapy,[20] and as a tool for predicting patient outcomes.[21–24] Despite these promising data, $^{18}$F-FDG evaluation in the brain has many challenges and limitations. For example, tumors located in or around regions of gray matter are difficult to delineate because of the intrinsically high $^{18}$F-FDG uptake in normal cortex. Additionally, studies have shown that only high-grade gliomas tend to be hypermetabolic on $^{18}$F-FDG PET, whereas low-grade gliomas can be isometabolic or even hypometabolic compared with surrounding tissue.[25] Furthermore, studies have shown that $^{18}$F-FDG uptake is not only confined to tumor cell metabolism but may also be confounded by stromal or inflammatory cell metabolism.[26] Together, these limitations have reduced enthusiasm for the routine use of $^{18}$F-FDG PET in brain tumor evaluation, resulting in investigations into other potentially valuable radiotracers.

### Amino Acid Tracers

An alternative target for molecular imaging of brain tumors involves labeling amino acids involved in protein metabolic pathways. Amino acid transport is increased in malignant cells,[27,28] which is hypothesized to be caused by the net result of increased demand for amino acids from amino acid synthesis for proliferation,[29,30] transamination, and transmethylation,[31,32] the use of amino acids as glutamine for fuel,[33] and as precursors for other biochemical syntheses. Regardless of the specific end use of these amino acids in brain tumors, various studies have shown that a wide variety of radiolabeled amino acids are useful for brain tumor molecular imaging. These tracers include [$^{11}$C-methyl]-methionine ($^{11}$C-MET), the most widely studied amino acid tracer in brain tumors to date,[34–36] L-1-[$^{11}$C]-tyrosine ($^{11}$C-TYR),[37–39] and other amino acids using the longer half-life [$^{18}$F] radiolabel including O-(2-[$^{18}$F]-fluoroethyl)-L-tyrosine ($^{18}$F-FET)[40–45] and 3,4-dihydroxy-6-[$^{18}$F]-fluoro-L-phenylalanine ($^{18}$F-FDOPA)[29,46–50] (and the $^{18}$F-FDOPA metabolite 3-O-methyl-6-[$^{18}$F]-fluoro-L-DOPA[51]). Although each of these amino acid tracers are unique in the complexity of their synthesis and their precise involvement in protein synthesis and amino acid uptake pathways, numerous studies have demonstrated that they have very similar patterns of abnormal tracer uptake and performance in identifying regions of active tumor.[44,46,52] Despite these promising results, amino acid uptake can also be elevated in inflammatory processes, such as sarcoidosis[53] and brain abscesses,[54] and it may be difficult to differentiate recurrent tumor from background tissue in many cases.[47]

## Proliferation Tracers

Investigations have clearly identified an indirect relationship between tumor proliferation rate and abnormal amino acid uptake in human brain tumors[29,30]; however, thymidine analogs (2-[$^{11}$C]-thymidine[55] or 3′-deoxy-3′-[$^{18}$F]-fluorothymidine [$^{18}$F-FLT][56]) allow for more direct quantification of proliferation rates through expression of the enzyme thymidine kinase-1 during DNA synthesis.[57] Numerous investigations have verified the strong correlation between $^{18}$F-FLT uptake parameters and brain tumor cell proliferation rates[57–59]; however, sensitivity seems to be somewhat limited.[60] Additionally, $^{18}$F-FLT tracers have higher variability in standard uptake value (SUV) uptake in normal white matter tissue,[61] potentially making it difficult to discern low-grade tumor proliferation from background activity. These challenges, along with a relatively difficult synthesis process, have limited the use of $^{18}$F-FLT to certain academic and research institutions.

## Hypoxia Tracers

When brain tumors proliferate they often outgrow their blood supply, resulting in a decrease in oxygen availability and localized hypoxia. This change in oxygen availability results in a variety of biologic responses, many of which are mediated by hypoxia-inducible factor, resulting in transcription of various target genes involved in angiogenesis, invasion, cell survival, and glucose metabolism.[62] As such, hypoxia is closely associated with brain tumor progression and treatment resistance.[63] [$^{18}$F]-fluoromisonidazole ($^{18}$F-FMISO) is a radiolabeled nitroimidazole derivative that can be used for PET imaging of tumor hypoxia[64,65] by trapping the metabolites within hypoxic cells.[66] Although not yet used in the clinic, $^{18}$F-FMISO has been shown to differentiate high- and low-grade gliomas,[67] has shown early promise as a biomarker for monitoring hypoxia changes during radiochemotherapy[68] and antiangiogenic therapy,[69] and may provide insight into patient outcomes.[70] Despite these promising initial findings, many factors currently limit the use of $^{18}$F-FMISO as a robust biomarker, including high background activity and relatively nonspecific uptake in low-grade gliomas.

## THE PET PARAMETRIC RESPONSE MAP

Evaluation of brain tumor response to therapy using PET is traditionally performed by quantifying the SUV, or kinetic properties, of the particular tracer within a specifically defined region of interest. For example, the mean $^{18}$F-FDG SUV within the contrast-enhancing tumor regions on postcontrast T1-weighted MR images has shown to be useful for evaluating brain tumors.[9] Although this method of tumor evaluation may be adequate for homogeneous solid or nodule lesions in other body organs, brain tumors are genetically and histopathologically heterogeneous leading to highly variable levels of uptake throughout the tumor regions. As such, simple evaluation using the mean or maximum uptake within a region of interest as a biomarker for tumor response may be inadequate because one area of the tumor may be responding to a particular therapy, whereas another region may be resistant to treatment and continuing to grow. To overcome the challenges associated with tumor heterogeneity, investigators have developed a method for quantifying the voxel-wise, or spatially specific, response to therapy termed "parametric response mapping" (PRMs).

The first applications of the PRM technique were in diffusion MR imaging data, when it was then termed "functional diffusion mapping."[71–75] Subsequently, this same methodology has been applied to quantify regional changes in cerebral blood volume using perfusion MR imaging,[76,77] changes in T2 relaxation rate on multiecho T2-weighted MR images,[78] and recently changes in $^{18}$F-FLT and $^{18}$F-FDOPA uptake.[61] Although the image signal of interest is different in each of these examples, the basic methodology of PRM generation and quantification is relatively similar.

### PET PRM Methodology

In general, PET PRMS are calculated by performing voxel-wise subtraction between tracer uptake on a follow-up PET scan during treatment and a baseline, or pretreatment, PET scan after aligning them both to the same image space (Fig. 1). First, follow-up PET scans (see Fig. 1A) are aligned with the follow-up anatomic MR images (see Fig. 1B). Similarly, baseline PET scans (see Fig. 1C) are aligned with the baseline anatomic MR images (see Fig. 1D). Because of the intrinsically low spatial resolution of PET scans, performing image alignment between PET scans on subsequent days is likely to impose substantial errors in registration. Instead, the anatomic MR images on follow-up (or posttreatment) (see Fig. 1E) are first registered to the baseline (or

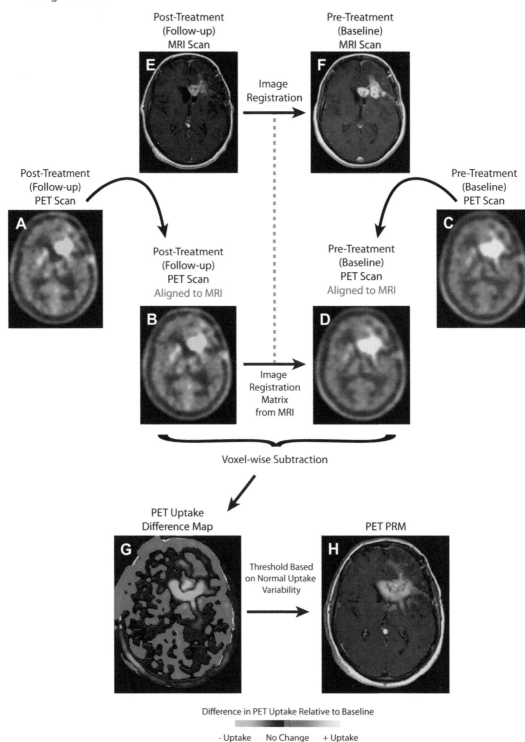

Fig. 1. PET PRM methodology. Calculation of PET PRMs begins with alignment of posttreatment (follow-up) PET scans (*A*) with posttreatment (follow-up) MR images before registration (*E*), resulting in registered posttreatment (follow-up) PET scans (*B*). Similarly, pretreatment (baseline) PET scans (*C*) are aligned with pretreatment (baseline) MR images before registration (*F*), resulting in registered pretreatment (baseline) PET scans (*D*). Posttreatment (follow-up) MR images (*E*) are then registered to pretreatment (baseline) MR images (*F*). The MR imaging–aligned PET scans (*B, D*) are then registered using the same image registration matrix calculated for the anatomic MR images (*E* and *F*). Voxel-wise subtraction is then performed, resulting in a PET uptake difference map (*G*). The final PET PRMs (*H*) are then generated by thresholding the PET uptake difference maps using information about the normal variability in PET uptake.

pretreatment) anatomic MR images (see **Fig. 1F**). Next, using the registration matrix calculated after alignment of the MR images, all follow-up PET scans are allineated with baseline PET scans. After alignment of all PET scans into the same image space, voxel-wise subtraction between subsequent follow-up PET scans and the baseline scans is performed (see **Fig. 1G**). Alternatively, the percentage change in PET uptake can be evaluated between subsequent PET scans with respect to a baseline scan. Finally, using a threshold for difference in tracer uptake based on empiric data related to the normal voxel-wise variability in PET uptake, only voxels that are outside this normal variation are considered "significantly different" and are retained in the final PET PRMs (see **Fig. 1H**).

### Threshold for PET PRM Classification Using Voxel-Wise Variation in PET Uptake

For PET PRMs to label voxels that have significant changes in tracer uptake between time points it is important to establish a normal range of uptake values that might be encountered during similar acquisition parameters. Traditionally, the range of acceptable values is determined by the 95% confidence interval for voxel-wise change in tracer uptake within normal-appearing tissue. This is done by first calculating PET SUV maps, then performing coregistration between two different time points within the same patient, and then performing voxel-wise subtraction of SUV values between these two time points (see **Fig. 1A–G**). After this is performed, the difference in SUV values within normal-appearing brain tissue (eg, normal-appearing, contralateral white matter) is extracted and used to estimate normal variation in PET uptake within this tissue. For example, **Fig. 2A–C** show histograms of voxel-wise change in $^{18}$F-FDOPA, $^{18}$F-FLT, and $^{18}$F-FDG uptake from pooled voxels from 5 to 10 patients within normal-appearing white matter. Results here suggest a 95% confidence interval for change in tracer uptake within normal-appearing white matter of 0.14, 0.62, and 0.14, respectively. Alternatively, the percentage change in uptake within normal brain tissue can be used, which was estimated around 14% for $^{18}$F-FDOPA and 30% for $^{18}$F-FLT.[61] Only voxels with a difference in uptake beyond these confidence intervals are considered a significant change in uptake and are retained for subsequent PRM analysis.

### Quantification of PET PRMs

There are many potential parameters that can be quantified through the use of PET PRMs.

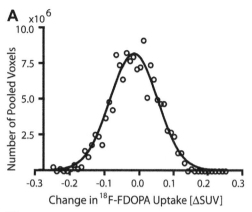

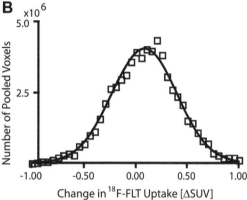

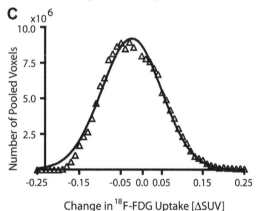

Fig. 2. Voxelwise variability in $^{18}$F-FDOPA, $^{18}$F-FLT, and $^{18}$F-FDG PET uptake within normal-appearing brain matter in patients with brain tumor. As a first estimate of the normal variation in SUV, the voxelwise variability in normal-appearing white matter was estimated for (A) $^{18}$F-FDOPA (N = 10 patients), (B) $^{18}$F-FLT (N = 10 patients), and (C) $^{18}$F-FDG (N = 5 patients).

Traditionally, the "volume fraction" of increasing or decreasing parameter values, defined as the percentage of a tumor region of interest (eg, contrast-enhancing or T2 hyperintense) with significantly increasing or decreasing parameter values ($\%Vol_{increasing}$, $\%Vol_{decreasing}$, $\%Vol_{changing}$), are used as the primary metrics for PRM evaluation. This approach, however, has the drawback of being highly dependent on initial tumor size. Alternatively, the absolute volume of tissue with significantly increasing or decreasing parameter values within a tumor region of interest or within the entire brain can be used ($Vol_{increasing}$, $Vol_{decreasing}$, $Vol_{changing}$). Other less widely used methods of PRM quantification include examining the distribution of voxelwise uptake changes, quantifying the mean or median voxelwise change in uptake within a tumor region of interest, or maximum contiguous cluster size with increasing or decreasing uptake.

## PET PRMS AS A BIOMARKER FOR EARLY TREATMENT RESPONSE

Although the PRM technique has been used in a variety of imaging modalities, there has only been a single study using PET PRMs,[61] with the purpose of evaluating early response to antiangiogenic therapy. The use of PET PRMs as a tool for detecting early treatment response is the most straightforward application, involving simply the voxel-wise subtraction of the posttreatment PET uptake values from the pretreatment values. Areas of the tumor that demonstrate a significant decrease in tracer uptake are thought to be regionally responding to treatment, whereas areas of the tumor that illustrate significant increases in tracer uptake are thought to be not responding to therapy. In this way, each patient's tumor may have regions that are responding to therapy and other areas where treatment is perhaps less effective.

Figs. 3 and 4 illustrate the [18]F-FDOPA and [18]F-FLT PET PRMs in a patient with a right temporal lobe glioblastoma that was treated with the antiangiogenic agent bevacizumab. Standard MR imaging showed a modest, but sustained radiographic response. Specifically, the volume of contrast-enhancement and T2 hyperintensity were only slightly reduced when evaluated at the first follow-up time point (4 weeks); however, by the second follow-up time point (8 weeks) the volume of contrast-enhancement and T2 hyperintensity were both reduced suggesting this patient may be responding to treatment. Interestingly, standard [18]F-FDOPA SUV maps suggest the volume of abnormal uptake may actually be increasing by the first follow-up time point, whereas reducing to the original tumor metabolic level by the second posttreatment follow-up time point. [18]F-FDOPA PRMs were able to clearly quantify the increase in [18]F-FDOPA uptake throughout the entire pretreatment contrast-enhancing tumor regions by the first follow-up time point; however,

when comparing the first with the second follow-up time point the amount of uptake was dramatically reduced. [18]F-FLT, however, was greatly reduced at both the first and the second follow-up time relative to the pretreatment baseline time point. This pattern of response was also captured by the [18]F-FLT PET PRMs, which indicated a significant reduction in [18]F-FLT uptake in the posteriomedial aspect of the tumor and a slight increase in uptake in the anteriolateral regions. [18]F-FLT PET PRMs showed further decrease in uptake between the first and second follow-up time points in the posterior regions of the tumor, but additional increase in uptake in the anterior, temporal pole regions.

[18]F-FDOPA and [18]F-FLT PET PRMs have recently demonstrated the ability to predict survival in patients treated with the antiangiogenic drug bevacizumab[61]; however, the sensitivity and specificity for each tracer, along with the particular PET PRM parameter with the best performance, varied dramatically similar to the results shown in Figs. 3 and 4. The absolute volume of tissue within contrast-enhancing regions of interest significantly increasing and decreasing in [18]F-FDOPA uptake after the first treatment with bevacizumab was found to be a significant predictor of 3-month progression-free survival (75% sensitivity and 70% specificity), whereas the volume fraction of contrast-enhancing tissue with significant increase in [18]F-FDOPA uptake between the first and second follow-up PET scans were predictive of 6-month overall survival in patients with recurrent malignant gliomas (91% sensitivity and 83% specificity). Alternatively, the volume fraction of contrast-enhancing tissue with either an increase or decrease in [18]F-FLT uptake after the first treatment of bevacizumab was a significant predictor of 3-month progression-free survival (90% sensitivity and 70% specificity) and the absolute volume of tissue with an increase in [18]F-FLT uptake after the first treatment of bevacizumab was a significant predictor of 6-month overall survival (75% sensitivity and 80% specificity). Together, these two sets of PET PRMs demonstrate the heterogeneity of response to therapy, and regional differences in the response dependent on the particular tracer being used.

PET PRMs can also be used to quantify response to therapy by evaluating the change in [18]F-FDG uptake. Figs. 5 and 6 show two patients with glioblastoma that were scanned before and after being placed on a new chemotherapeutic, having failed standard therapy. For one patient (see Fig. 5), standard postcontrast T1-weighted MR images show a growing enhancing mass in the left temporal lobe after being placed on

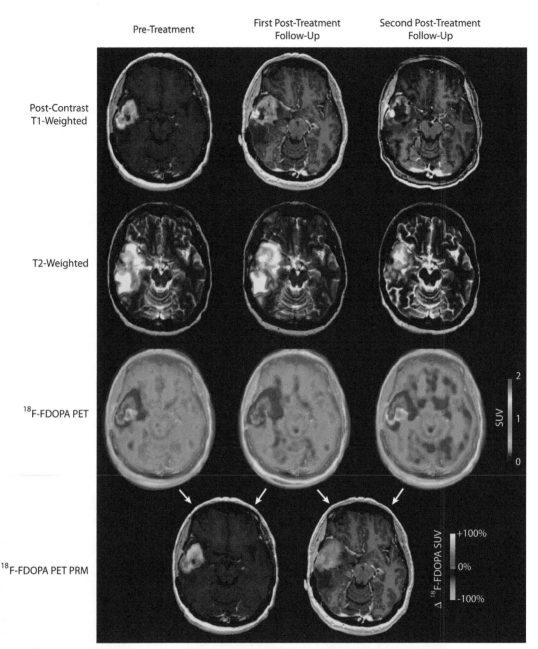

**Fig. 3.** $^{18}$F-FDOPA PET PRMs in a patient with glioblastoma treated with bevacizumab. (*Top Row*) Postcontrast, T1-weighted MR images before (*left column*), at the first follow-up time point (*middle column*), and the second follow-up time point (*right column*). (*Second Row*) T2-weighted images before, at first follow-up, and at second follow-up. (*Third Row*) $^{18}$F-FDOPA PET SUV maps at each time point. (*Bottom Row*) Calculated $^{18}$F-FDOPA PET PRMs for the pretreatment and first posttreatment PET scan (*left PRM*) and first and second follow-up PET scans (*right PRM*).

therapy. Emission scans for $^{18}$F-FDG show elevated glucose uptake in the left temporal pole before and after therapy, and a slightly smaller mass with abnormal uptake after therapy. Contradictory to the MR imaging observations, $^{18}$F-FDG PET PRMs demonstrated widespread decrease in uptake throughout the entire enhancing lesion, with a slightly larger decrease in uptake in the posterior aspect of the tumor, suggesting this increase in contrast enhancement may be more related to treatment effects than growing tumor.

**Fig. 6** illustrates the response of another patient with glioblastoma to the same chemotherapy treatment paradigm, but with a different response

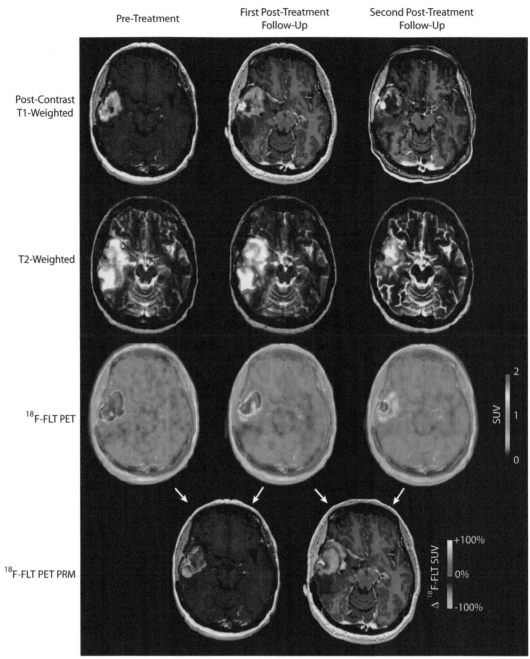

Pre-Treatment

First Post-Treatment
Follow-Up

Second Post-Treatment
Follow-Up

Post-Contrast
T1-Weighted

T2-Weighted

$^{18}$F-FLT PET

$^{18}$F-FLT PET PRM

SUV

$\Delta$ $^{18}$F-FLT SUV

Fig. 4. $^{18}$F-FLT PET PRMs in a patient with glioblastoma treated with bevacizumab. (*Top Row*) Postcontrast, T1-weighted MR images before (*left column*), at the first follow-up time point (*middle column*), and the second follow-up time point (*right column*). (*Second Row*) T2-weighted images before, at first follow-up, and at second follow-up. (*Third Row*) $^{18}$F-FLT PET SUV maps at each time point. (*Bottom Row*) Calculated $^{18}$F-FLT PET PRMs for the pretreatment and first posttreatment PET scan (*left PRM*) and first and second follow-up PET scans (*right PRM*).

on $^{18}$F-FDG PET PRMs. Standard postcontrast T1-weighted images showed a slightly larger volume of contrast enhancement after initiation of therapy. Emission scans for $^{18}$F-FDG show

lower uptake in the tumor regions compared with surrounding cortex, which is a known limitation of $^{18}$F-FDG. After therapy, $^{18}$F-FDG emission scans appeared similar to those obtained

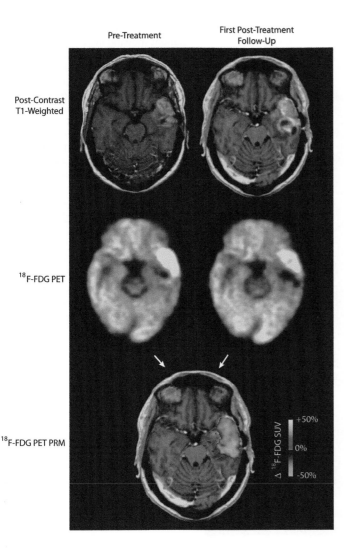

Pre-Treatment

First Post-Treatment
Follow-Up

Post-Contrast
T1-Weighted

$^{18}$F-FDG PET

$^{18}$F-FDG PET PRM

+50%

0%

-50%

$\Delta$ $^{18}$F-FDG SUV

**Fig. 5.** $^{18}$F-FDG PET PRM in a patient showing decreased uptake after treatment, but a growing contrast-enhancing lesion. (*Top Row*) Postcontrast, T1-weighted MR images before (*left column*) and after (*right column*) a new treatment after recurrence. (*Middle Row*) $^{18}$F-FDG PET emission scans before and after treatment. (*Bottom Row*) Calculated $^{18}$F-FDG PET PRMs illustrating decreased uptake despite an increase in contrast enhancement.

pretreatment, providing little insight into whether metabolic changes within the tumor have occurred as a result of therapy. $^{18}$F-FDG PET PRMs, however, demonstrated more than a 50% increase in glucose uptake relative to pretreatment levels in the anterior portion of the tumor, suggesting the increase in contrast enhancement, in this case, was likely caused by growing tumor and not as a result of successful treatment.

Quantitative treatment response evaluation is the most straightforward application of the PET PRM technique. Examination of voxel-wise changes in PET tracer uptake between pretreatment and posttreatment time points allows for regional response to be measured and visualized in individual patients. Although this technique has currently been implemented in only a single study involving two tracers, PET PRMs have the potential to play an important role in testing novel treatments in the clinic.

## PET PRMS FOR SERIAL CLINICAL MONITORING

Another powerful application of PET PRMs involves quantitatively monitoring tumor growth in patients over time. Although standard, static emission tomographic images can be used to evaluate whether or not a lesion has abnormal uptake, serial registration of PET scans and evaluations with respect to a single time point allows for more subtle changes in uptake to be detected. This is of particular importance for low-grade tumors that grow relatively slowly over the course of many years.

**Fig. 7** illustrates this concept in a patient with low-grade mixed oligodendroglioma with a very slow-growing tumor. In 2008, this patient first received a gross total resection of a nonenhancing right frontal lobe tumor and received 24 cycles of temozolomide, a cytotoxic chemotherapeutic.

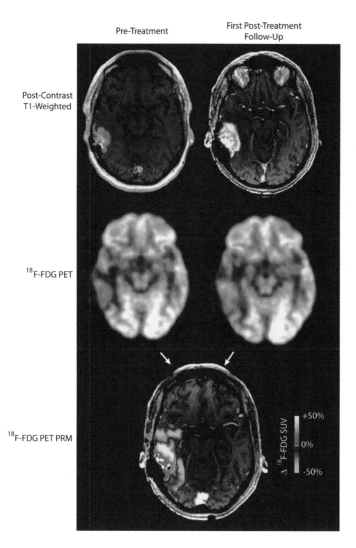

Pre-Treatment

First Post-Treatment
Follow-Up

Post-Contrast
T1-Weighted

$^{18}$F-FDG PET

$^{18}$F-FDG PET PRM

Fig. 6. $^{18}$F-FDG PET PRM in a patient showing increased uptake after treatment, but a growing contrast-enhancing lesion. (*Top Row*) Postcontrast, T1-weighted MR images before (*left column*) and after (*right column*) a new treatment after recurrence. (*Middle Row*) $^{18}$F-FDG PET emission scans before and after treatment. (*Bottom Row*) Calculated $^{18}$F-FDG PET PRMs illustrating increased uptake along with an increase in contrast enhancement.

MR imaging and $^{18}$F-FDOPA PET scans were obtained in 2009, 2011, and in 2012, but no substantial changes in anatomic or molecular images were noted during this period. Specifically, T2 hyperintensity on fluid-attenuated inversion recovery images shows a nodular lesion in the posterior aspect of the resection cavity, which corresponds spatially to the region with elevated $^{18}$F-FDOPA uptake that appears relatively stable over time. $^{18}$F-FDOPA PET PRMs, however, clearly show continual growth of this tumor over time when evaluated with respect to the 2008 PET scans in medial aspect of the resection cavity adjacent to the nodule thought to harbor the growing tumor. In this way, PET PRMs may provide quantitative information about the direction of tumor spread independent of changes in MR imaging or static PET scans.

Although the use of a single, fixed scan session as a baseline can be advantageous for detecting subtle changes in tumor metabolism over time, often many different treatments are used at different time points during each patient's course of therapy, thereby obscuring interpretation of PET PRMs depending on the baseline time point used. Therefore, the use of a "moving baseline" form of PET PRMs can also be of clinical value. Fig. 8 shows PET PRMs generated in a 52-year-old male patient with a left-sided low-grade mixed oligodendroglioma. Baseline $^{18}$F-FDOPA PET scans were obtained in February 2010, during a course of treatment with the alkylating chemotherapeutic lomustine. The patient later finished treatment and was no longer on adjuvant therapy. At the time of the second $^{18}$F-FDOPA PET scan the patient was suspected of tumor recurrence. $^{18}$F-FDOPA PET PRMs evaluated between these two time points clearly identified a region of increased $^{18}$F-FDOPA uptake in the left internal capsule, adjacent to the lateral ventricles. This patient was

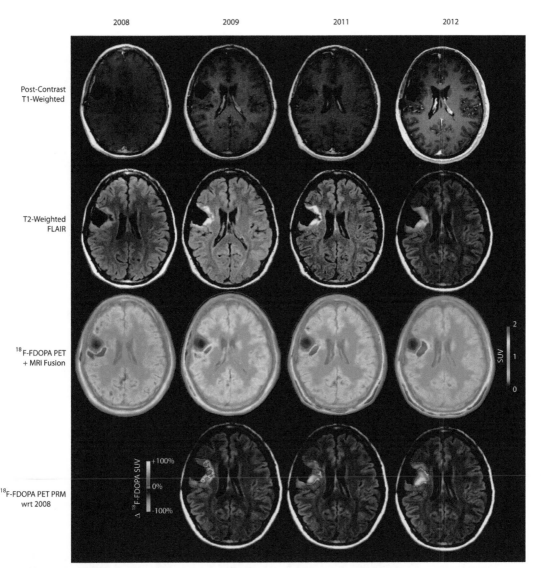

**Fig. 7.** $^{18}$F-FDOPA PET PRMs for clinical monitoring of a patient with low-grade glioma. (*Top Row*) Postcontrast, T1-weighted MR images during long-term follow-up. (*Second Row*) T2-weighted MR images during long-term follow-up. (*Third Row*) $^{18}$F-FDOPA PET SUV maps during long-term follow-up. (*Bottom Row*) Calculated $^{18}$F-FDOPA PET PRMs illustrating growing tumor over time.

then put on bevacizumab, an antiangiogenic agent, combined with carboplatin, a cytotoxic chemotherapeutic. In February 2012, the patient received a third $^{18}$F-FDOPA PET scan for a possible recurrence on bevacizumab. $^{18}$F-FDOPA PET PRMs were then constructed between the previous time point, in November 2010, and the most recent scans to determine whether $^{18}$F-FDOPA uptake was elevated with respect to pre-bevaciumab levels. $^{18}$F-FDOPA PET PRMs verified that the region in the internal capsule had decreased $^{18}$F-FDOPA uptake; however, regions near the cortex had elevated uptake similar to the scans from February 2010. In this way,

"moving baseline" PET PRMs helped to provide additional information about subtle changes in tracer uptake between sequential PET scans, instead of a single fixed baseline time point, in a patient with a complex treatment history.

## TECHNICAL LIMITATIONS OF PET PRMS

Despite the apparent advantages of using PET PRMs to quantify treatment response and monitor tumor growth, there are a few technical limitations that should be considered. First, PET PRM performance may be dependent on the accuracy of image registration between different time points;

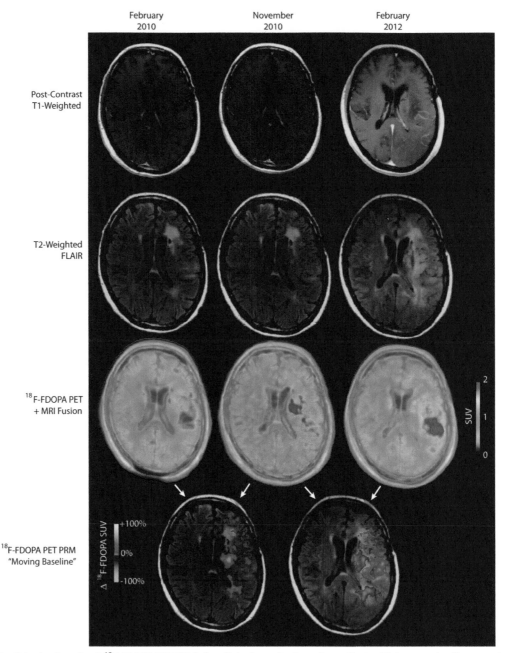

**Fig. 8.** "Moving baseline" [18]F-FDOPA PET PRMs for clinical monitoring of a patient with low-grade glioma on two different treatments during follow-up. (*Top Row*) Postcontrast, T1-weighted MR images during long-term follow-up. (*Second Row*) T2-weighted MR images during long-term follow-up. (*Third Row*) [18]F-FDOPA PET SUV maps during long-term follow-up. (*Bottom Row*) Calculated "moving baseline" [18]F-FDOPA PET PRMs illustrating growing tumor at different time points using a different (moving) pretreatment baseline.

however, PET PRMs are likely less sensitive to misregistration compared with PRMs generated from MR imaging techniques because of the inherently lower resolution of PET scans. If this misregistration is caused by mass effect from either growing tumor or reduction in edema from antiangiogenic therapy, then nonlinear (elastic)

registration of the anatomic MR images may be useful, as was demonstrated in a previous study involving functional diffusion mapping (diffusion PRMs).[79]

**Fig. 9** demonstrates how nonlinear warping of anatomic MR imaging data to compensate for mass effect may be performed for PET PRMs in

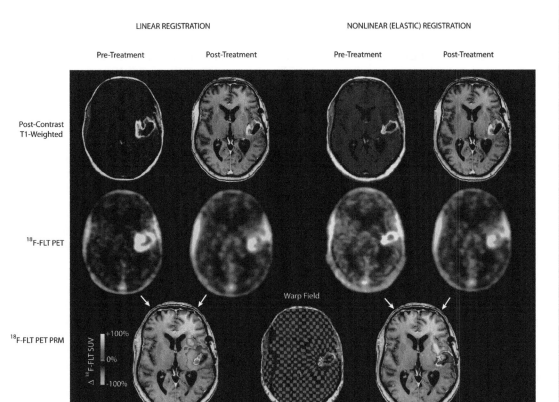

**Fig. 9.** Linear and nonlinear (elastic) registration of anatomic MR imaging data to correct [18]F-FLT PET PRMs for mass effect. (*Left Two Columns*) Linear registration. (*Right Two Columns*) Nonlinear (elastic) registration of the pretreatment to posttreatment time point. (*Top Row*) Postcontrast, T1-weighted images pretreatment (*left*) and posttreatment (*right*). (*Middle Row*) [18]F-FLT PET emission scans pretreatment (*left*) and posttreatment (*right*). (*Bottom Row*) [18]F-FLT PET PRMs after linear registration (*far left*) and nonlinear registration (*far right*). Also shown is the warp field used to nonlinearly register MR images, which was later applied to the PET scans for nonlinear PET PRMs.

a patient with recurrent glioblastoma treated with bevacizumab. As illustrated by the postcontrast T1-weighted images (*left*), the patient had a reduction in the cystic cavity volume after treatment with bevaiczumab resulting in the entire brain shifting back toward relatively normal anatomic position. [18]F-FLT emission scans show elevated proliferation on the rim of the lesion and residual elevated [18]F-FLT uptake after therapy, although the lesion itself appears smaller because of reduction in the cystic necrotic cavity volume. If [18]F-FLT PET PRMs are performed for these two time points using linear registration then the lesion looks like it responded because the highly proliferative, contrast-enhancing rim is misaligned between the subsequent time points. Alternatively, if nonlinear registration is used to align the pretreatment [18]F-FLT PET scans to the posttreatment [18]F-FLT scans using the registration matrix from the anatomic, postcontrast T1-weighted images, the resulting [18]F-FLT PET PRMs are dramatically

different. In particular, the contrast-enhancing region of the tumor only shows a modest decrease in uptake, whereas the highly proliferative nodule on the anteriomedial portion of the lesion did not have a significant change in [18]F-FLT uptake, consistent with qualitative observations of the emission scans. Nonlinear registration techniques applied to PET scans for generation of PRMs need more testing to confirm their use.

A few more potential limitations warrant a brief discussion. First, lag between the timing of the PET and anatomic MR images used for image registration could pose a potential confound to PET PRM interpretation. If PET scans are not obtained simultaneously (ie, using a combined MR-PET system), or if PET scans were obtained on different days than the MR examination, there is potential for slight misalignment of the anatomy between the PET and MR images because of tumor growth or mass effect. A second possible confound to interpretation of PET PRMs is the lack of accounting for the time between subsequent PET scans. For example, if one patient receives subsequent PET scans 2 weeks apart and another patient receives subsequent PET scans 2 months apart, but both show the same degree of change in tracer uptake, traditional PET PRMs would be interpreted as having a similar response regardless of how fast or slow it may have occurred. One simple solution to this limitation may be to divide the resulting PET PRMs by the time interval between PET scans, resulting in maps that quantify the "time rate of change in tracer uptake." Finally, PET PRMs may be confounded by changes in corticosteroid dose that occur during the course of treatment, so it is important to interpret PET PRMs with caution because changes in corticosteroid dose can change vascular permeability that, in some cases, can change the apparent tracer uptake.

## FUTURE DIRECTIONS

PET PRMs are a new technique for clinically monitoring tumor growth and quantifying treatment response; however, they have not been fully explored or validated. Therefore, many avenues of research and technical improvements may exist. For example, PET PRMs could be applied during radiotherapy to monitor response to treatment and perhaps boost radiation dose to areas that appear less responsive. The use of more advanced registration techniques or temporal compensation may further improve performance of PET PRMs. Exploring PET PRMs applied to pharmacokinetic parameters extracted from dynamic PET data instead of SUV may also be of added value, because many tracers are dependent on vascular permeability and may be confounded by changes in steroid dose. Perhaps most importantly, PET PRMs need validation of spatial accuracy through the use of stereotactic biopsy to confirm that regions deemed not responsive truly represent growing tumor.

## SUMMARY

PET PRMs are a provocative new method for quantifying tumor response to therapy in individual patients. By aligning sequential PET scans over time, the voxel-wise change in radiotracer uptake can be quantified and visualized, which is particularly beneficial for highly heterogeneous malignant brain tumors where part of the tumor may respond to therapy, whereas another portion may not. PET PRMs can be performed before and after a particular therapy to test whether the tumor is responding favorably. Alternatively, PET PRMs can be

performed relative to a distant time point to monitor changes through the course of a treatment. Future studies aimed at testing this technique with various radiotracers and therapies, along with technical improvements, are warranted.

## REFERENCES

1. CBTRUS Statistical Report: Primary Brain and Central Nervous System Tumors Diagnosed in the United States in 2004–2006. Hinsdale (IL): Central Brain Tumor Registry of the United States; 2010. Available at: www.cbtrus.org.
2. Stupp R, Mason WP, van den Bent MJ, et al. Radiotherapy plus concomitant and adjuvant temozolomide for glioblastoma. N Engl J Med 2005;352:987.
3. Macdonald DR, Cascino TL, Schold SC Jr, et al. Response criteria for phase II studies of supratentorial malignant glioma. J Clin Oncol 1990;8:1277.
4. Wen PY, Macdonald DR, Reardon DA, et al. Updated response assessment criteria for high-grade gliomas: response assessment in neuro-oncology working group. J Clin Oncol 2010;28:1963.
5. Di Chiro G, DeLaPaz RL, Brooks RA, et al. Glucose utilization of cerebral gliomas measured by [18F] fluorodeoxyglucose and positron emission tomography. Neurology 1982;32:1323.
6. Di Chiro G. Positron emission tomography using [18F] fluorodeoxyglucose in brain tumors. A powerful diagnostic and prognostic tool. Invest Radiol 1987;22:360.
7. Gambhir SS, Czernin J, Schwimmer J, et al. A tabulated summary of the FDG PET literature. J Nucl Med 2001;42:1S.
8. Hustinx R, Smith RJ, Benard F, et al. Can the standardized uptake value characterize primary brain tumors on FDG-PET? Eur J Nucl Med 1999;26:1501.
9. Kosaka N, Tsuchida T, Uematsu H, et al. 18F-FDG PET of common enhancing malignant brain tumors. AJR Am J Roentgenol 2008;190:W365.
10. Kahn D, Follett KA, Bushnell DL, et al. Diagnosis of recurrent brain tumor: value of 201Tl SPECT vs. 18F-fluorodeoxyglucose PET. AJR Am J Roentgenol 1994;163:1459.
11. Kim EE, Chung SK, Haynie TP, et al. Differentiation of residual or recurrent tumors from post-treatment changes with F-18 FDG PET. Radiographics 1992; 12:269.
12. Langleben DD, Segall GM. PET in differentiation of recurrent brain tumor from radiation injury. J Nucl Med 2000;41:1861.
13. Stokkel M, Stevens H, Taphoorn M, et al. Differentiation between recurrent brain tumour and post-radiation necrosis: the value of 201Tl SPET versus 18F-FDG PET using a dual-headed coincidence camera–a pilot study. Nucl Med Commun 1999;20:411.

14. Thompson TP, Lunsford LD, Kondziolka D. Distinguishing recurrent tumor and radiation necrosis with positron emission tomography versus stereotactic biopsy. Stereotact Funct Neurosurg 1999;73:9.

15. Delbeke D, Meyerowitz C, Lapidus RL, et al. Optimal cutoff levels of F-18 fluorodeoxyglucose uptake in the differentiation of low-grade from high-grade brain tumors with PET. Radiology 1995;195:47.

16. Kincaid PK, El-Saden SM, Park SH, et al. Cerebral gangliogliomas: preoperative grading using FDG-PET and 201TI-SPECT. AJNR Am J Neuroradiol 1998;19:801.

17. Ericson K, Kihlstrom L, Mogard J, et al. Positron emission tomography using 18F-fluorodeoxyglucose in patients with stereotactically irradiated brain metastases. Stereotact Funct Neurosurg 1996; 66(Suppl 1):214.

18. Rozental JM, Cohen JD, Mehta MP, et al. Acute changes in glucose uptake after treatment: the effects of carmustine (BCNU) on human glioblastoma multiforme. J Neurooncol 1993;15:57.

19. Valk PE, Budinger TF, Levin VA, et al. PET of malignant cerebral tumors after interstitial brachytherapy. Demonstration of metabolic activity and correlation with clinical outcome. J Neurosurg 1988;69:830.

20. Colavolpe C, Chinot O, Metellus P, et al. FDG-PET predicts survival in recurrent high-grade gliomas treated with bevacizumab and irinotecan. Neuro Oncol 2012;14:649.

21. De Witte O, Lefranc F, Levivier M, et al. FDG-PET as a prognostic factor in high-grade astrocytoma. J Neurooncol 2000;49:157.

22. Pardo FS, Aronen HJ, Fitzek M, et al. Correlation of FDG-PET interpretation with survival in a cohort of glioma patients. Anticancer Res 2004;24:2359.

23. Spence AM, Muzi M, Graham MM, et al. 2-[(18)F] Fluoro-2-deoxyglucose and glucose uptake in malignant gliomas before and after radiotherapy: correlation with outcome. Clin Cancer Res 2002;8: 971.

24. Tralins KS, Douglas JG, Stelzer KJ, et al. Volumetric analysis of 18F-FDG PET in glioblastoma multiforme: prognostic information and possible role in definition of target volumes in radiation dose escalation. J Nucl Med 2002;43:1667.

25. Padma MV, Said S, Jacobs M, et al. Prediction of pathology and survival by FDG PET in gliomas. J Neurooncol 2003;64:227.

26. Kubota R, Yamada S, Kubota K, et al. Intratumoral distribution of fluorine-18-fluorodeoxyglucose in vivo: high accumulation in macrophages and granulation tissues studied by microautoradiography. J Nucl Med 1992;33:1972.

27. Busch H, Davis JR, Honig GR, et al. The uptake of a variety of amino acids into nuclear proteins of tumors and other tissues. Cancer Res 1959;19:1030.

28. Isselbacher KJ. Sugar and amino acid transport by cells in culture: differences between normal and malignant cells. N Engl J Med 1972;286:929.

29. Kato T, Shinoda J, Oka N, et al. Analysis of 11C-methionine uptake in low-grade gliomas and correlation with proliferative activity. AJNR Am J Neuroradiol 2008;29:1867.

30. Sato N, Suzuki M, Kuwata N, et al. Evaluation of the malignancy of glioma using 11C-methionine positron emission tomography and proliferating cell nuclear antigen staining. Neurosurg Rev 1999; 22:210.

31. Chiang PK, Cantoni GL. Activation of methionine for transmethylation. Purification of the S-adenosylmethionine synthetase of bakers' yeast and its separation into two forms. J Biol Chem 1977;252:4506.

32. Meyer GJ, Schober O, Hundeshagen H. Uptake of 11C-L- and D-methionine in brain tumors. Eur J Nucl Med 1985;10:373.

33. Souba WW. Glutamine and cancer. Ann Surg 1993; 218:715.

34. Bergstrom M, Collins VP, Ehrin E, et al. Discrepancies in brain tumor extent as shown by computed tomography and positron emission tomography using [68Ga]EDTA, [11C]glucose, and [11C]methionine. J Comput Assist Tomogr 1983;7:1062.

35. Ericson K, Lilja A, Bergstrom M, et al. Positron emission tomography with ([11C]methyl)- L-methionine, [11C]D-glucose, and [68Ga]EDTA in supratentorial tumors. J Comput Assist Tomogr 1985;9:683.

36. Lilja A, Bergstrom K, Hartvig P, et al. Dynamic study of supratentorial gliomas with L-methyl-11C-methionine and positron emission tomography. AJNR Am J Neuroradiol 1985;6:505.

37. Go KG, Keuter EJ, Kamman RL, et al. Contribution of magnetic resonance spectroscopic imaging and L-[1-11C]tyrosine positron emission tomography to localization of cerebral gliomas for biopsy. Neurosurgery 1994;34:994.

38. Heesters MA, Go KG, Kamman RL, et al. 11C-tyrosine position emission tomography and 1H magnetic resonance spectroscopy of the response of brain gliomas to radiotherapy. Neuroradiology 1998;40:103.

39. Willemsen AT, van Waarde A, Paans AM, et al. In vivo protein synthesis rate determination in primary or recurrent brain tumors using L-[1-11C]-tyrosine and PET. J Nucl Med 1995;36:411.

40. Dunet V, Rossier C, Buck A, et al. Performance of 18F-fluoro-ethyl-tyrosine (18F-FET) PET for the differential diagnosis of primary brain tumor: a systematic review and Metaanalysis. J Nucl Med 2012;53:207.

41. Pauleit D, Floeth F, Hamacher K, et al. O-(2-[18F] fluoroethyl)-L-tyrosine PET combined with MRI improves the diagnostic assessment of cerebral gliomas. Brain 2005;128:678.

42. Popperl G, Gotz C, Rachinger W, et al. Value of O-(2-[18F]fluoroethyl)- L-tyrosine PET for the diagnosis of recurrent glioma. Eur J Nucl Med Mol Imaging 2004;31:1464.

43. Rachinger W, Goetz C, Popperl G, et al. Positron emission tomography with O-(2-[18F]fluoroethyl)-L-tyrosine versus magnetic resonance imaging in the diagnosis of recurrent gliomas. Neurosurgery 2005;57:505.

44. Weber WA, Wester HJ, Grosu AL, et al. O-(2-[18F]fluoroethyl)-L-tyrosine and L-[methyl-11C]methionine uptake in brain tumours: initial results of a comparative study. Eur J Nucl Med 2000;27:542.

45. Wester HJ, Herz M, Weber W, et al. Synthesis and radiopharmacology of O-(2-[18F]fluoroethyl)-L-tyrosine for tumor imaging. J Nucl Med 1999;40:205.

46. Becherer A, Karanikas G, Szabo M, et al. Brain tumour imaging with PET: a comparison between [18F]fluorodopa and [11C]methionine. Eur J Nucl Med Mol Imaging 2003;30:1561.

47. Fueger BJ, Czernin J, Cloughesy T, et al. Correlation of 6-18F-fluoro-L-dopa PET uptake with proliferation and tumor grade in newly diagnosed and recurrent gliomas. J Nucl Med 2010;51:1532.

48. Heiss WD, Wienhard K, Wagner R, et al. F-Dopa as an amino acid tracer to detect brain tumors. J Nucl Med 1996;37:1180.

49. Ledezma CJ, Chen W, Sai V, et al. 18F-FDOPA PET/MRI fusion in patients with primary/recurrent gliomas: initial experience. Eur J Radiol 2009;71:242.

50. Schiepers C, Chen W, Cloughesy T, et al. 18F-FDOPA kinetics in brain tumors. J Nucl Med 2007;48:1651.

51. Beuthien-Baumann B, Bredow J, Burchert W, et al. 3-O-methyl-6-[18F]fluoro-L-DOPA and its evaluation in brain tumour imaging. Eur J Nucl Med Mol Imaging 2003;30:1004.

52. Grosu AL, Astner ST, Riedel E, et al. An interindividual comparison of O-(2-[18F]fluoroethyl)-L-tyrosine (FET)- and L-[methyl-11C]methionine (MET)-PET in patients with brain gliomas and metastases. Int J Radiat Oncol Biol Phys 2011;81:1049.

53. Yamada Y, Uchida Y, Tatsumi K, et al. Fluorine-18-fluorodeoxyglucose and carbon-11-methionine evaluation of lymphadenopathy in sarcoidosis. J Nucl Med 1998;39:1160.

54. Floeth FW, Pauleit D, Sabel M, et al. 18F-FET PET differentiation of ring-enhancing brain lesions. J Nucl Med 2006;47:776.

55. Eary JF, Mankoff DA, Spence AM, et al. 2-[C-11] thymidine imaging of malignant brain tumors. Cancer Res 1999;59:615.

56. Chen W, Cloughesy T, Kamdar N, et al. Imaging proliferation in brain tumors with 18F-FLT PET: comparison with 18F-FDG. J Nucl Med 2005;46:945.

57. Rasey JS, Grierson JR, Wiens LW, et al. Validation of FLT uptake as a measure of thymidine kinase-1 activity in A549 carcinoma cells. J Nucl Med 2002;43:1210.

58. Backes H, Ullrich R, Neumaier B, et al. Noninvasive quantification of 18F-FLT human brain PET for the assessment of tumour proliferation in patients with high-grade glioma. Eur J Nucl Med Mol Imaging 2009;36:1960.

59. Ullrich R, Backes H, Li H, et al. Glioma proliferation as assessed by 3'-fluoro-3'-deoxy-L-thymidine positron emission tomography in patients with newly diagnosed high-grade glioma. Clin Cancer Res 2008;14:2049.

60. Schwarzenberg J, Czernin J, Cloughesy TF, et al. 3'-deoxy-3'-18F-fluorothymidine PET and MRI for early survival predictions in patients with recurrent malignant glioma treated with bevacizumab. J Nucl Med 2012;53:29.

61. Harris RJ, Cloughesy TF, Pope WB, et al. 18F-FDOPA and 18F-FLT positron emission tomography parametric response maps predict response in recurrent malignant gliomas treated with bevacizumab. Neuro Oncol 2012;14:1079–89.

62. Kaur B, Khwaja FW, Severson EA, et al. Hypoxia and the hypoxia-inducible-factor pathway in glioma growth and angiogenesis. Neuro Oncol 2005;7:134.

63. Brown JM. Therapeutic targets in radiotherapy. Int J Radiat Oncol Biol Phys 2001;49:319.

64. Rasey JS, Koh WJ, Evans ML, et al. Quantifying regional hypoxia in human tumors with positron emission tomography of [18F]fluoromisonidazole: a pretherapy study of 37 patients. Int J Radiat Oncol Biol Phys 1996;36:417.

65. Valk PE, Mathis CA, Prados MD, et al. Hypoxia in human gliomas: demonstration by PET with fluorine-18-fluoromisonidazole. J Nucl Med 1992;33:2133.

66. Whitmore GF, Varghese AJ. The biological properties of reduced nitroheterocyclics and possible underlying biochemical mechanisms. Biochem Pharmacol 1986;35:97.

67. Hirata K, Terasaka S, Shiga T, et al. (1)(8)F-Fluoromisonidazole positron emission tomography may differentiate glioblastoma multiforme from less malignant gliomas. Eur J Nucl Med Mol Imaging 2012;39:760.

68. Narita T, Aoyama H, Hirata K, et al. Reoxygenation of glioblastoma multiforme treated with fractionated radiotherapy concomitant with temozolomide: changes defined by 18F-fluoromisonidazole positron emission tomography: two case reports. Jpn J Clin Oncol 2012;42:120.

69. Valable S, Petit E, Roussel S, et al. Complementary information from magnetic resonance imaging and (18)F-fluoromisonidazole positron emission tomography in the assessment of the response to an anti-angiogenic treatment in a rat brain tumor model. Nucl Med Biol 2011;38:781.

70. Spence AM, Muzi M, Swanson KR, et al. Regional hypoxia in glioblastoma multiforme quantified with [18F]fluoromisonidazole positron emission tomography before radiotherapy: correlation with time to progression and survival. Clin Cancer Res 2008;14:2623.

71. Ellingson BM, Cloughesy TF, Lai A, et al. Graded functional diffusion map-defined characteristics of apparent diffusion coefficients predict overall survival in recurrent glioblastoma treated with bevacizumab. Neuro Oncol 2011;13:1151.

72. Ellingson BM, Cloughesy TF, Zaw T, et al. Functional diffusion maps (fDMs) evaluated before and after radiochemotherapy predict progression-free and overall survival in newly diagnosed glioblastoma. Neuro Oncol 2012;14:333.

73. Ellingson BM, Malkin MG, Rand SD, et al. Validation of functional diffusion maps (fDMs) as a biomarker for human glioma cellularity. J Magn Reson Imaging 2010;31:538.

74. Moffat BA, Chenevert TL, Lawrence TS, et al. Functional diffusion map: a noninvasive MRI biomarker for early stratification of clinical brain tumor response. Proc Natl Acad Sci U S A 2005;102:5524.

75. Moffat BA, Chenevert TL, Meyer CR, et al. The functional diffusion map: an imaging biomarker for the early prediction of cancer treatment outcome. Neoplasia 2006;8:259.

76. Galban CJ, Chenevert TL, Meyer CR, et al. The parametric response map is an imaging biomarker for early cancer treatment outcome. Nat Med 2009; 15:572.

77. Tsien C, Galban CJ, Chenevert TL, et al. Parametric response map as an imaging biomarker to distinguish progression from pseudoprogression in high-grade glioma. J Clin Oncol 2010;28:2293.

78. Ellingson BM, Cloughesy TF, Lai A, et al. Quantification of edema reduction using differential quantitative T2 (DQT2) relaxometry mapping in recurrent glioblastoma treated with bevacizumab. J Neurooncol 2012;106:111.

79. Ellingson BM, Cloughesy TF, Lai A, et al. Nonlinear registration of diffusion-weighted images improves clinical sensitivity of functional diffusion maps in recurrent glioblastoma treated with bevacizumab. Magn Reson Med 2012;67: 237.

# Novel Quantitative Techniques in Hybrid (PET-MR) Imaging of Brain Tumors

Srinivasan Senthamizhchelvan, PhD[a],
Habib Zaidi, PhD, PD[b,c,d],*

## KEYWORDS

- PET • MRI • Hybrid imaging • Quantification • Radiation therapy • Image segmentation

## KEY POINTS

- Multimodality imaging has become an integral part in the medical management of brain tumors for the past 2 decades.
- Hybrid PET-MR technology is a major breakthrough and offers many quantitative avenues for brain tumor assessment and quantification.
- In radiation oncology, image-guided patient-specific treatment planning has become a standard practice, making use of high-precision dose-delivery techniques.
- The success of image-guided radiotherapy is directly related to the accuracy of imaging methods in distinguishing tumors from surrounding normal tissues, which makes PET-MR an essential imaging modality.
- Studying tumor biology at the molecular level using PET-MR will help in charting personalized treatment plans for patients with a brain tumor and also in exploring new therapeutic opportunities in the future.

## INTRODUCTION

Brain tumors are a collection of heterogeneous intracranial neoplasms, each with its own biology, treatment, and prognosis.[1] Although magnetic resonance (MR) imaging is the best imaging option for diagnosing brain tumors, understanding tumor biology at the molecular level is essential for early detection and also for delivering effective personalized treatments. Positron emission tomography (PET) is one of the most prominent molecular imaging modalities used for imaging pathophysiology of tumors at an early stage. Currently, no single imaging modality can provide the sensitivity, specificity, and high spatial resolution required in distinguishing brain tumors from surrounding normal tissues. Hence, combining anatomic and functional imaging modalities has been explored to achieve the stated goals. So far, hybrid technologies, including PET–computed tomography (CT) and PET-MR have successfully been used for brain tumor management in clinics. The quest for combined multimodality imaging is an ongoing process. In a recent study, combining MR, photoacoustics, and Raman imaging has been shown to provide promising results in identifying brain tumor margins in animal models.[2]

PET-MR has shown to be superior to CT, PET, or MR alone, mainly because it allows for molecular, anatomic, and functional imaging with uncompromised quality.[3] Tumor delineation using

[a] The Russell H. Morgan Department of Radiology and Radiological Science, Johns Hopkins University School of Medicine, Baltimore, MD, USA; [b] Division of Nuclear Medicine and Molecular Imaging, Geneva University Hospital, CH-1211 Geneva, Switzerland; [c] Geneva Neuroscience Center, Geneva University, CH-1211 Geneva, Switzerland; [d] Department of Nuclear Medicine and Molecular Imaging, University Medical Center Groningen, University of Groningen, 9700 RB Groningen, The Netherlands
* Corresponding author. Division of Nuclear Medicine, Geneva University Hospital, CH-1211 Geneva, Switzerland.
E-mail address: habib.zaidi@hcuge.ch

PET Clin 8 (2013) 219–232
http://dx.doi.org/10.1016/j.cpet.2012.09.007
1556-8598/13/$ – see front matter Published by Elsevier Inc.

the PET component with the help of high-resolution MR has proved to be advantageous compared with the use of a single modality, given the complementary information provided by each one. Imaging amino acid transport using PET tracers plays a potentially important clinical role in brain tumor detection.[4] [18]F-fluoro-ethyl-tyrosine ([18]F-FET) PET demonstrated excellent results in diagnosing primary brain tumors.[5] Biologic brain tumor target volume has shown to be defined more accurately and rationally when [11]C-choline PET is combined with MR imaging.[6] It has been shown that [11]C-choline PET has a higher sensitivity and specificity in distinguishing recurrent brain tumors from radionecrosis compared with [18]F-fluoro-deoxy-glucose ([18]F-FDG) PET and MR imaging.[7] The diagnostic accuracy can benefit from coregistration of PET and MR imaging, enabling the fusion of high-resolution morphologic images with corresponding biologic information. Software-based multimodality image registration for the brain has been shown to be robust and accurate and is being routinely used in the clinic for various applications, including tumor imaging.[8] These procedures are further optimized on dedicated PET-MR, systems permitting the simultaneous assessment of morphologic, functional, metabolic, and molecular information on the human brain.[9,10] In this report, we review the recent advances and clinical applications of quantitative PET-MR in brain tumor imaging.

## ADVANCES IN HYBRID PET-MR INSTRUMENTATION FOR BRAIN IMAGING
### From the Limited Role of CT in PET-CT to the Promise of MR in PET-MR

The introduction of combined PET-CT scanners was an instant game changer in medical imaging and has superseded standalone PET scanners. Integrated PET-CT scanners allowed the overlay of sequentially acquired CT and PET images and have been a practical and viable approach in obtaining coregistered functional and anatomic images in a single scanning session. However, for brain imaging, the poor soft tissue contrast of CT has long been a drawback. This has been one of the compelling reasons for integrating high-resolution anatomic information from MR imaging with the functional PET information. Initially, intra-modality image registration methods were used and were found to be inadequate, which prompted the idea of simultaneous PET-MR prototypes for animal imaging.[11] PET has very high sensitivity for tracking biomarkers in vivo but has poor resolving power for morphology, whereas MR imaging has lower sensitivity, but produces high soft tissue

contrast. Combining PET and MR imaging in a single platform to harness the synergy of these 2 modalities is very intuitive and logical. The synergy of PET-MR has proven very powerful in studying biology and pathology in the preclinical setting and has great potential for clinical applications.[12] A typical example in which PET-MR plays a key role over PET-CT is illustrated in **Fig. 1.** PET-MR overcomes many limitations of PET-CT, such as limited tissue contrast and high radiation doses delivered to the patient or the animal being studied.[13] In addition, recent PET-MR designs allow for simultaneous rather than sequential acquisition of PET and MR imaging data, which could not have been achieved through a combination of PET and CT scanners.[14]

### Dedicated Brain PET-MR Instrumentation

Hybrid PET-MR technology was initially developed for imaging small animal models of human disease,[11,12,15,16] and through many years of technical improvements was shown to be feasible in imaging the human brain[17,18] and the whole body.[14,19] Combining PET and MR for simultaneous acquisition of spatially and temporally correlated PET-MR data sets is technically challenging owing to the strong magnetic fields in the MR subsystem. Despite the challenges and technical difficulties, a clinical PET-MR prototype (BrainPET, Siemens Medical Solutions, Erlangen, Germany) dedicated for simultaneous PET-MR brain imaging was developed and installed in a few institutions for validation and testing.[17] The system was assessed in clinical and research settings in 5 academic institutions in Germany and the Unites States by exploiting the full potential of anatomic MR imaging in terms of high soft tissue contrast sensitivity in addition to the many other possibilities offered by this modality, including blood oxygenation level–dependent imaging, functional MR imaging, diffusion-weighted imaging, perfusion-weighted imaging, and diffusion tensor imaging.[20] A second sequential combined PET-MR system was also designed for molecular-genetic brain imaging by docking separate PET and MR systems together so that they share a common bed that passes through the field of view of both cameras.[21] This was achieved by combining 2 high-end imaging devices, namely a high-resolution research tomograph and a 7-T MR image with submillimeter resolution.

Dedicated PET-MR is a valuable tool for grading of brain tumors, detection of recurrences, and monitoring treatment response. MR imaging alone is not sufficient in applications, such as defining tumor infiltration boundaries and therapy response evaluation wherein biologic changes precede

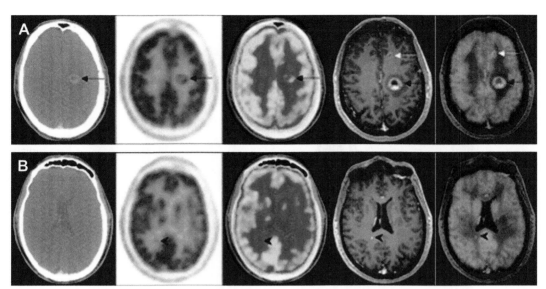

Fig. 1. A 54-year-old patient with cerebral metastases from cancer of unknown primary. (*A*) Large left-hemisphere metastasis (*black arrow*) is visible on (from left to right) axial contrast-enhanced CT, [18]F-FDG PET, PET-CT, axial contrast-enhanced MR imaging, and PET/MR imaging, whereas smaller metastasis of left frontal lobe (*white arrow*) is visible solely on MR imaging and PET/MR imaging. Location of this metastasis directly adjacent to highly [18]F-FDG–avid cortex leads to problems with diagnosing this lesion on [18]F-FDG PET scan. (*B*) Another subcentimeter-sized metastasis of right temporal lobe, clearly visible on MR imaging and PET/MR imaging of same patient (*arrowhead*), was only retrospectively seen as faintly increased [18]F-FDG activity on [18]F-FDG PET and PET-CT because of lack of anatomic correlate on CT. (*Adapted from* Buchbender C, Heusner TA, Lauenstein TC, et al. Oncologic PET/MRI, Part 1: tumors of the brain, head and neck, chest, abdomen, and pelvis. J Nucl Med 2012;53(6):928–38; with permission.)

morphologic signals. **Fig. 2** shows representative clinical brain PET-CT and PET-MR images of a healthy subject acquired sequentially on 2 combined systems, namely the Biograph TrueV (Siemens Healthcare, Erlangen, Germany)[22] and Ingenuity TF PET-MRI (Philips Healthcare, Eindhoven, The Netherlands).[19] The PET-CT study was started 30 minutes following injection of 370 MBq of [18]F-FDG followed by PET-MR imaging, which started about 80 minutes later. The better soft tissue contrast observed on MR imaging is obvious and further emphasizes the ineffectiveness of PET-CT for this indication and the potential role of PET-MR imaging.[23,24]

## INNOVATIONS IN MR IMAGING–GUIDED QUANTITATIVE BRAIN PET IMAGING

PET-MR imaging has primarily been used to fuse functional/molecular and anatomic data to facilitate anatomic localization of functional abnormalities and also to aid in quantitative analysis of specific regions of interest or at the voxel level. In addition, anatomic information derived from MR imaging might also be useful for attenuation correction, motion compensation, scatter modeling and correction, and partial volume correction and could

serve as *a priori* information to guide the PET reconstruction process. In spite of the widespread interest in PET-MR imaging, there are several challenges that face the use of PET-MR in clinical settings.

## MR Imaging–Guided Attenuation Correction in PET-MR

Quantitative measurement of PET radiotracer activity concentration requires correction for photon attenuation and much of PET-MR success in the future will likely depend on the accuracy of determining an attenuation map from the MR signal. Because of space constraints, a transmission scan system can hardly be fit inside a PET-MR scanner, although a recent study reported on the placement of an annulus Ge-68 transmission source inside the field of view of the PET detector ring, thus enabling simultaneous acquisition of 511-keV photons emanating from the patient and the transmission source.[25] Time-of-flight information is used to discriminate the coincident photons originating from the transmission source. Unlike PET-CT, attenuation correction in PET-MR systems is not trivial because the MR signal reflects tissue proton densities and relaxation times and

**PET-CT**

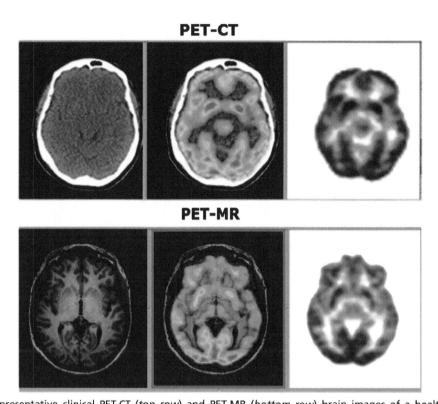

**PET-MR**

Fig. 2. Representative clinical PET-CT (*top row*) and PET-MR (*bottom row*) brain images of a healthy subject acquired sequentially (~80-minute time difference) on 2 combined systems (Siemens Biograph TrueV and Philips Ingenuity TF PET-MRI, respectively) following injection of 370 MBq of $^{18}$F-FDG. (*Courtesy of* Geneva University Hospital.)

not electron density. Moreover, MR signals are not directly related to the tissue attenuation.[26] This becomes a limiting issue in locating and mapping bone, brain skull, lungs, and other unpredictable benign or malignant anatomic abnormalities with varying densities. Bone is intrinsically not detectable by conventional MR sequences, as it shows up as a black or void region, which makes it difficult to distinguish bone from air. In the head, however, the skull bone is covered by subcutaneous fat and encloses the brain. Incorporation of *a priori* anatomic knowledge allows for sufficient information to be collected to precisely segment MR scans and thus to provide an accurate attenuation map.

Various approaches have been used to derive the attenuation map from MR images.[27] Segmentation of gray matter, white matter, and water equivalent soft tissue structures are relatively trivial but it is highly challenging to segment bone tissue from air-filled spaces using conventional MR sequences. Zaidi and colleagues[28] have developed an MR-guided attenuation correction technique for brain PET imaging to alleviate the requirement of acquiring an x-ray CT scan using fuzzy logic segmentation. Using segmented T1-weighted 3-dimensional MR images, the

investigators have shown the possibility of deriving a nonuniform attenuation map from MR imaging for brain PET imaging. The procedure was further refined by automating the segmentation of the skull procedure of T1-weighted MR image using a sequence of mathematical morphologic operations.[29] A proof of principle of the use of dual-echo ultra-short echo time MR imaging–based attenuation correction in brain imaging to discriminate air-filled cavities from bone on MR images was also reported.[30,31]

An alternative to the image segmentation approach is the use of anatomic atlas registration for attenuation correction where the PET atlas is registered to the patient's PET and prior knowledge of the atlas' attenuation properties is used to build a patient-specific attenuation map.[32] Deformable image registration plays a key role in atlas-based attenuation correction, which may fail in situations with large deformations. Moreover, it is not clear to what extent global anatomy from an atlas could realistically predict an individual patient's attenuation map. Hofmann and colleagues[33] studied an MR-guided attenuation correction technique using image segmentation and a method based on an atlas registration and pattern recognition (AT&PR) algorithm in 11 patients and reported that the MR-guided technique using AT&PR provided better overall PET quantification accuracy than the basic MR image segmentation approach because of the significantly reduced volume of errors made regarding volumes of interest within or near bones and the slightly reduced volume of errors made regarding areas outside the lungs. Marshall and colleagues[34] developed a technique wherein variable lung density was taken into account in the attenuation correction of whole-body PET-MR imaging. The investigators first established a relationship between MR imaging and CT signal in the lungs and used it to predict attenuation coefficients from MR imaging. They reported that their technique improved the quantitative fidelity of PET images in the lungs and nearby tissues compared with an approach that assumes uniform lung density. Recently, Chang and colleagues[35] investigated the use of

nonattenuated PET images as a means for attenuation correction of PET images in PET-MR systems using a 3-step iterative process and suggested that the technique is feasible in the clinics and can potentially be an alternative method of MR-based attenuation correction in PET-MR imaging.

Fig. 3 illustrates different ways of deriving the attenuation map for brain PET imaging including transmission scanning, model or atlas-based approaches, x-ray CT, segmented T1-weighted MR imaging, and more sophisticated MR imaging–guided derivation of the attenuation map. Fig. 3 also shows the transaxial CT cross section, the corresponding coregistered MR imaging cross section, and the segmented MR image required in generating a 3-tissue compartment head model corresponding to brain, skull, and scalp using the algorithm mentioned previously.[36] Compensation for attenuation in the bed and head holder can be accomplished as

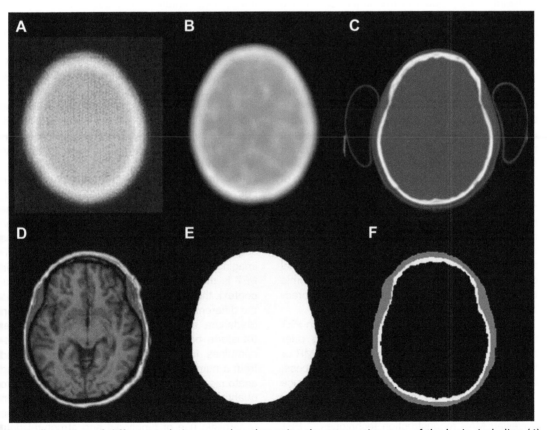

Fig. 3. Illustration of different techniques used to determine the attenuation map of the brain, including (A) model-based techniques producing a 3-class attenuation map, (B) transmission scan, (C) X-ray CT transaxial cross section and its corresponding coregistered MR imaging cross section (D), the segmented MR imaging required to generate a single-class (E) by thresholding and 3-class compartment head model corresponding to brain, skull and scalp. (F) White voxels are labeled as skull, dark gray voxels are labeled as scalp, and intracranial black voxels are labeled as brain tissue.

discussed previously for calculated attenuation correction methods.[29]

Many challenging issues, such as contrast insta- bility of MR in comparison with CT, inaccuracies associated with assigning theoretical or uniform attenuation coefficients, motion artifacts, and attenuation of MR hardware, still need to be addressed adequately.[24] MR-guided attenuation correction is clearly evolving and will remain a hot topic that requires further research and development efforts. Apparent other advantages of MR are in motion correction and in partial volume correction of PET data.

### MR Imaging–Guided PET Image Reconstruction and Partial Volume Correction

Statistical methods have been increasingly used in PET image reconstruction because of their better noise properties. In addition, information regarding the image formation and physics processes can be incorporated using Bayesian *priors*. However, an undesirable by-product of the statistical iterative reconstruction techniques, such as maximum likelihood-expectation maximization algorithm (ML-EM), is that large numbers of iterations are prone to increase the noise content of the recon- structed PET images. In emission tomography, photon noise is modeled as having a Poisson distri- bution. The noise characteristics can be overcome by incorporating *a priori* distribution to describe the statistical properties of the unknown image and thus produce *a posteriori* probability distributions from the image conditioned on the data. Bayesian reconstruction methods form a logical extension of the ML-EM algorithm. Maximization of the *a poste- riori* (MAP) probability over the set of possible images results in the MAP estimate. This approach has many advantages, as various components of the prior, such as pseudo-Poisson nature of statis- tics, non-negativity of the solution, local voxel correlations, or known existence of anatomic boundaries may be added individually in the prac- tical implementation of the algorithms.[37]

Using a Bayesian resolution loss model in PET images can be avoided by incorporating prior anatomic information from a coregistered MR or CT image in the PET reconstruction process. Combined PET-CT and PET-MR systems produce accurately registered anatomic and functional image data that can be exploited in developing Bayesian MAP reconstruction techniques.[38] PET image reconstruction using MAP has been shown to have improved contrast versus noise tradeoff.[39] In brain imaging, MR imaging–guided PET image reconstruction was reported to outperform CT- guided reconstruction owing to the high soft tissue

contrast provided by MR and the accuracy ob- tained using sophisticated brain MR imaging segmentation procedures.[40]

The quantitative accuracy of PET activity concentration estimates for sources having dimen- sions less than twice the system's spatial resolution is limited because the counts in smaller volumes are spread over a larger volume than the physical size of the object owing to the limited spatial reso- lution of the imaging system. This phenomenon is referred to as the partial volume effect (PVE) and can be corrected using one of the various strategies developed for this purpose. In multimodality brain imaging, a main concern has been related to the PVE correction for cerebral metabolism in the atro- phied brain, particularly in Alzheimer disease (AD). The accuracy of MR imaging–guided PVE correc- tion in PET largely depends on the accuracy achieved by the PET-MR imaging coregistration procedure, which is improved by using simulta- neous hybrid PET-MR imaging systems. Zaidi and colleagues[40] evaluated the impact of brain MR image segmentation methods on PET partial volume correction in [18]F-FDG and [18]F-L-dihydrox- yphenylalanine ([18]F-DOPA) brain PET imaging. The results indicated that a careful choice of the segmentation algorithm should be made while using geometric transfer matrix–based partial volume corrections in brain PET.

Fig. 4 illustrates the impact of PVE correction in functional FDG-PET brain imaging of a patient with suspected AD.[23] The voxel-based MR imaging– guided PVE correction applied here follows the approach by Matsuda and colleagues.[41]

Recently, Wang and Fei[42] introduced a PVE correction method that incorporates edge informa- tion in MR imaging to guide PET partial volume correction without MR imaging segmentation taking advantage of the PET-MR alignment. The second issue affecting the accuracy of MR imaging–guided partial volume correction in brain PET is the MR segmentation procedure. In this context, the high soft tissue contrast of MR allows the differentiation between gray and white matter. Shidahara and colleagues[43] studied a wavelet transform–based synergistic approach that combines functional and structural information from a number of sources (CT, MR imaging, and anatomic probabilistic atlases) for the accurate quantitative recovery of radioactivity concentration in PET images. The study demonstrated that the synergistic use of functional and structural data yields morphologically corrected PET images of high quality. Le Pogam and colleagues[44] proposed a voxel-wise PVE correction based on the original mutual multiresolution analysis approach (MAA). The study showed an improved and more robust

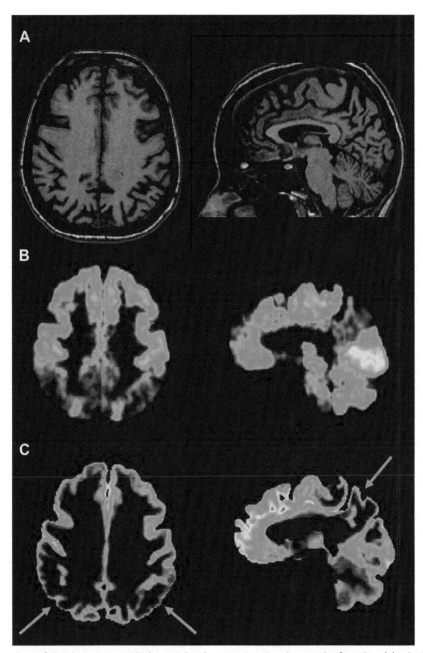

Fig. 4. Illustration of MR imaging–guided partial volume correction impact in functional brain PET imaging showing for a patient with probable Alzheimer's disease the original T1-weighted MR image (A) and PET image before (B) and after partial volume effect correction (C). The arrows put in evidence that the hypometabolism extends beyond the atrophy.

qualitative and quantitative accuracy compared with the MAA methodology, particularly in the absence of full correlation between anatomic and functional information.

## MR Imaging–Guided Motion Correction

The intrinsic spatial resolution achieved using high-resolution PET scanners available today does not translate into spatial resolution achieved in the clinical imaging because of various factors, including motion during or between the anatomic and functional image acquisitions.[45] Patient motion (voluntary or involuntary)–related quantitative inaccuracy is common in imaging the brain, head and neck, thoracic, and abdomen regions because of long PET acquisition time. Although the common misalignment between PET and CT images in the thoracic region on combined PET-CT scanners is related to differences between breathing patterns and acquisition times, this challenging issue will likely be addressed partly in some cases, but not necessarily in all, through the introduction of PET-MR because of the longer acquisition time of typical MR sequences used for attenuation correction, thus leading to temporal averaging and improvement in the alignment between MR imaging and PET.

In brain PET-MR prototype scanners, rigid-body[46] and nonrigid motion correction[47] methods have been successfully tested for improved spatial resolution and accurate PET quantification. Tsoumpas and colleagues[48] studied the potential of using MR-derived motion fields to correct nonrigid motion in PET and showed that combined PET-MR acquisitions could potentially allow motion compensation in whole-body PET acquisitions without prolonging acquisition time or increasing radiation dose. In neurologic simultaneous PET-MR studies, Catana and colleagues[49] showed, using 3-dimensional Hoffman brain phantom and human volunteer studies, that high temporal-resolution MR imaging–derived motion estimates acquired simultaneously on the hybrid brain PET-MR scanner can be used to improve PET image quality, therefore increasing its reliability, reproducibility, and quantitative accuracy. Imaging in vivo primates, Chun and colleagues[47] have recently shown that tagged MR imaging–based motion correction in simultaneous PET-MR significantly improves lesion detection compared with respiratory gating and no motion correction while reducing radiation dose.

## ROLE OF HYBRID PET-MR FOR TARGET VOLUME DELINEATION OF BRAIN TUMORS
### Rationale Behind the Use of PET in Biologic Tumor Volume Delineation

In radiotherapy treatment planning, the identification of gross tumor boundaries, known as gross tumor volume (GTV), is the first essential step. Knowledge of anatomic and functional tumor extent with respect to surrounding normal tissue is essential in GTV delineation. In brain tumors, the identification of aggressive tumor components within spatially heterogeneous lesions is challenging.[50] MR imaging allows precise information on tumor morphology but fails to provide details on tumor activity and metabolism. PET helps in tumor grading, assessing tumor extent, and in studying metabolism. As such, combined PET-MR reins in the synergy and helps in personalized radiotherapy treatment planning in brain tumors.[51]

In the radiotherapy treatment planning of glioblastoma multiforme (GBM), MR imaging is routinely used for GTV delineation. One of the caveats in using MR imaging for delineating glioma tumor boundaries is that MR imaging is unreliable mainly because of the inherently infiltration nature of GBM and the lack of distinction between glioma and surrounding edema with MR imaging. Increasing evidence suggests that brain tumor imaging with PET using amino acids is more reliable than MR imaging to define the extent of cerebral gliomas.[5,6,52] Fig. 5. is an example of the applicability and clinical usefulness of combined PET-MR in the imaging of brain tumors.

### PET Image Segmentation Techniques

Identifying a perfect image segmentation algorithm in the absence of the ground truth and considering the imperfect system response function is a challenge in PET quantification. In addition, the low spatial resolution and high noise characteristics of PET images makes image segmentation a difficult task. Image segmentation is defined as the process of classifying the voxels of an image into a set of distinct classes. Image segmentation has been identified as the key problem of medical image analysis and remains a challenging and fascinating area of research. Despite the difficulties and known limitations, several image segmentation approaches have been proposed and used in the clinical setting, including thresholding, region growing, classifiers, clustering, edge detection, Markov random field models, artificial neural networks, deformable models, atlas-guided, and many other approaches.[53]

Manual segmentation methods available on most commercial software packages to identify lesion boundaries and to quantify GTVs in terms of standardized uptake value are very laborious and tedious. They discourage physicians from taking advantage of the inherently quantitative data and compel them to use qualitative means in their diagnosis, therapy planning, and assessment of patient response to therapy. Semiautomated or fully automated segmentation methods enable physicians to easily extract maximum and mean standardized uptake value estimates from a lesion volume. This also allows the physician to track changes in lesion size and uptake after radio/chemotherapy. At present, various methods are used in practice to delineate PET-based target volumes.[53]

Manual delineation of target volumes using different window-level settings and look-up tables is the most common and widely used technique in the clinic; however, the method is highly

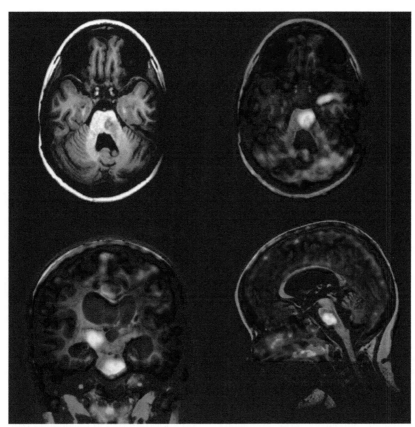

**Fig. 5.** Transaxial $^{18}$F-FET PET-MR images of a 7-year-old girl with carcinoma of the choroid plexus (*top row*). The exact localization of the tumors is pinpointed on the fused coronal/sagittal PET-MR images (*bottom row*). (*Courtesy of* Geneva University Hospital.)

operator-dependent and is subject to high variability among operators. Rather large intraobserver variability was reported[54] for many localizations, including high-grade glioma (HGG), as shown in **Fig. 6**. In this respect, semiautomated or fully automated delineation techniques might offer several advantages over manual techniques by reducing operator error/subjectivity, thereby improving reproducibility. Our group reported on the contribution of $^{18}$F-FET PET in the delineation of GTV in patients with HGG as compared with MR imaging alone using manual and semiautomated techniques.[55] In this study, PET-based tumor volumes were delineated in 18 patients using 7 image-segmentation techniques. The PET image-segmentation techniques included manual delineation of contours (GTV$_{(man)}$), a 2.5 standardized uptake value (SUV) cutoff (GTV$_{(2.5)}$), a fixed threshold of 40% and 50% of the maximum signal intensity (GTV$_{(40\%)}$ and GTV$_{(50\%)}$), signal-to-background ratio (SBR)-based adaptive thresholding (GTV$_{(SBR)}$), gradient find (GTV$_{(GF)}$), and region growing (GTV$_{(RG)}$). Overlap analysis was also conducted to assess geographic mismatch between the GTVs delineated using the different techniques. Contours defined using GTV$_{(2.5)}$ failed to provide successful delineation technically in 3 patients (18% of cases) as SUV(max) less than 2.5 and clinically in 14 patients (78% of cases). Overall, most GTVs defined on PET-based techniques were usually found to be smaller than GTV$_{(MR\ imaging)}$ (67% of cases). Yet, PET frequently detected tumors that were not visible on MR imaging and added substantial tumor extension outside the GTV$_{(MR\ imaging)}$ in 6 patients (33% of cases). The study showed that the selection of the most appropriate $^{18}$F-FET PET-based segmentation algorithm is crucial, as it affects both the volume and shape of the resulting GTV. The SBR-based PET technique was shown to be useful and suggested that it may add considerably important information on tumor extent to conventional MR imaging–guided GTV delineation.

## Amino Acids in Brain Gliomas

Amino acid (AA)-based PET tracers (AA-PET) L-methyl-[C-11]methionine (MET), and $^{18}$F-FET

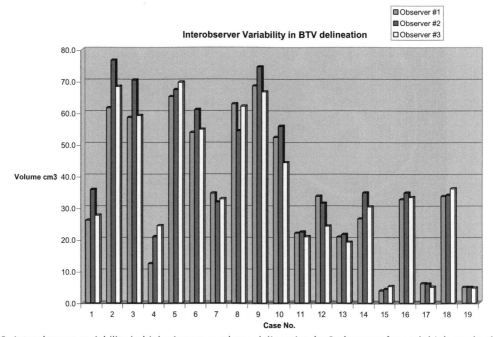

**Fig. 6.** Interobserver variability in biologic tumor volume delineation by 3 observers for each high-grade glioma case (1 through 19). (*Adapted from* Zaidi H, Senthamizhchelvan S. Assessment of biologic target volume using positron emission tomography in high-grade glioma patients. In: Hayat E, editor. Tumors of the central nervous system. vol. 2. New York: Springer; 2011:131–41.)

have shown higher sensitivity and specificity (85%–95%) for malignant gliomas in comparison with MR imaging. MET-PET and FET-PET have shown to have similar tumor uptake patterns.[56] AA-PET has been gaining interest and is routinely being performed to differentiate viable tumor form radiation-induced necrotic regions. In GTV delineation, AA-PET is used to determine tumor extent. Grosu and colleagues[57] showed the utility of MET-PET and iodo-methyl-tyrosine single-photon emission computed tomography (SPECT) for GTV delineation in gliomas. An increase in median survival from 6 months to 11 months has been reported in patients with recurrent high-grade gliomas whose radiotherapy treatment was planned on the basis of biologic imaging using MET-PET or SPECT in comparison with those patients whose treatment was planned conventionally.[58] Galldiks and colleagues[59] studied treatment response in patients with glioblastoma using [18]F-FET PET alongside MR imaging and showed that in comparison with MR imaging tumor volumes, changes in [18]F-FET PET may be a valuable parameter to assess treatment response in glioblastoma and to predict survival time. This study and other studies have exemplified the relevance of metabolically active tumor volumes in AA-PET to assess treatment response.[59,60] **Fig. 7** demonstrates a typical case in which PET plays

an important role in delineating biologically active tumor volume over MR alone.

## Other Relevant Tracers for Brain Tumor Imaging

Tumor hypoxia remains the most challenging condition for treatment. Although oxygen metabolism in gliomas differs from that of normal brain tissue, the lack of oxygen appears to be an important factor in determining glioma aggressiveness and response to therapy. It has been documented in several types of cancers that low levels of oxygen tension are associated with persistent tumor following radiation therapy and with the subsequent development of local recurrences. In gliomas, spontaneous necrosis suggests the presence of hypoxic regions that are radioresistant. Most of the PET tracers for tumor hypoxia are from the family of 2′-nitroimidazole compounds, which exhibit a rate of uptake that is purely dependent on the oxygen concentration.[61] Currently available hypoxia-imaging agents include, but not are limited to, [18]F-fluoroazomycinarabinofuranoside ([18]F-FAZA), and its iodinated counterparts ([123]I/[124]I-IAZA), [18]F-fluoromisonidazole ([18]F-MISO), [64]Cu-diacetyl-bis(N4-methylthiosemicarbazone) ([64]Cu-ATSM), or [99m]Tc-labeled and [68]Ga-labeled metronidazole. The role of hypoxia imaging in measuring the extent of tumor hypoxia,

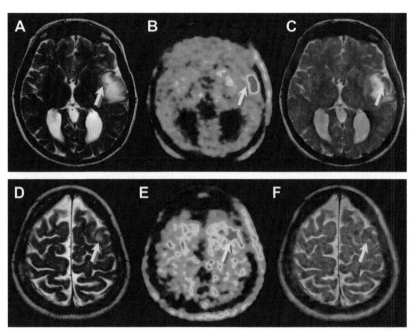

Fig. 7. Example of a patient with a glioblastoma (WHO IV) in the left temporal and frontal areas. The images shown on the *top row* (temporal area) correspond to gadolinium-enhanced T2-weighted MR imaging (*A*), coregistered [18]F-FET (*B*), and fused PET-MR (*C*) of the first study. The same is shown in the *bottom row* for the same study in the frontal area (*D–F*). The [18]F-FET PET study revealed an additional lesion missed on MR imaging. In addition, the T2-weighted MR imaging and the [18]F-FET PET show substantially different gross tumor volume extension for radiation therapy treatment planning. (*Adapted from* Zaidi H, Senthamizhchelvan S. Assessment of biologic target volume using positron emission tomography in high-grade glioma patients. In: Hayat E, editor. Tumors of the central nervous system. vol. 2. New York: Springer; 2011:131–41.)

and intratumoral special distribution of hypoxia are excellent for therapy decision making; however, it is worth mentioning that the tumor-to-blood ratio is generally low in hypoxia imaging, which may translate into statistical uncertainties in measuring intratumoral hypoxic regions.[62] PET imaging of tumor hypoxia has been identified as a prognostic biomarker.[63,64] In addition, the spatial distribution of hypoxic regions within the tumors can guide biologically based radiotherapy treatment planning.[65] In gliomas, there is increasing evidence that tumor hypoxia correlates with radioresistance and the extent of hypoxia in gliomas before radiotherapy is related to decrease in tumor progression time or patient survival time.[66,67] [18]F-FMISO imaging of hypoxic glioma cells shows significant promise; however, larger patient population studies are required to ascertain its clinical impact. Identifying the regional distribution of hypoxia may improve planning of resections and allow targeting higher doses of radiotherapy more precisely to the hypoxic areas.

## SUMMARY AND FUTURE PERSPECTIVES

Multimodality imaging has become an integral part in the medical management of brain tumors for the past 2 decades. Hybrid PET-MR technology is a major breakthrough and offers many quantitative avenues for brain tumor assessment and quantification. PET imaging provides the opportunity to image noninvasively many biologic processes. Regional biologic information and pathophysiology of brain tumors can be obtained by studying energy metabolism, AA transport, hypoxia, proliferation, and cell death. In radiation oncology, image-guided patient-specific treatment planning has become standard practice, making use of high-precision dose-delivery techniques; however, the success of image-guided radiotherapy is directly related to the accuracy of imaging methods in distinguishing tumors from surrounding normal tissues, which makes PET-MR an essential imaging modality. Studying tumor biology at the molecular level using PET-MR will help in charting personalized treatment plans for patients with brain tumors and also in exploring new therapeutic opportunities in the future.

## ACKNOWLEDGMENTS

This work was supported by the Swiss National Science Foundation under grants SNSF

31003A-125246, 33CM30-124114, Geneva Cancer League, and the Indo-Swiss Joint Research Program ISJRP 138866.

## REFERENCES

1. DeAngelis LM. Brain tumors. N Engl J Med 2001; 344(2):114–23.
2. Kircher MF, de la Zerda A, Jokerst JV, et al. A brain tumor molecular imaging strategy using a new triple-modality MRI-photoacoustic-raman nanoparticle. Nat Med 2012;18(5):829–U235.
3. Schwenzer NF, Stegger L, Bisdas S, et al. Simultaneous PET/MR imaging in a human brain PET/MR system in 50 patients—current state of image quality. Eur J Radiol 2012;81(11):3472–8.
4. Walter F, Cloughesy T, Walter MA, et al. Impact of 3,4-Dihydroxy-6-18F-Fluoro-L-Phenylalanine PET/CT on managing patients with brain tumors: the referring physician's perspective. J Nucl Med 2012; 53(3):393–8.
5. Dunet V, Rossier C, Buck A, et al. Performance of 18F-fluoro-ethyl-tyrosine (18F-FET) PET for the differential diagnosis of primary brain tumor: a systematic review and metaanalysis. J Nucl Med 2012;53(2): 207–14.
6. Li FM, Nie Q, Wang RM, et al. (11)C-CHO PET in optimization of target volume delineation and treatment regimens in postoperative radiotherapy for brain gliomas. Nucl Med Biol 2012;39(3):437–42.
7. Tan H, Chen L, Guan Y, et al. Comparison of MRI, F-18 FDG, and 11C-choline PET/CT for their potentials in differentiating brain tumor recurrence from brain tumor necrosis following radiotherapy. Clin Nucl Med 2011;36(11):978–81.
8. Slomka P, Baum R. Multimodality image registration with software: state-of-the-art. Eur J Nucl Med Mol Imaging 2009;36(Suppl 1):44–55.
9. Heiss WD, Raab P, Lanfermann H. Multimodality assessment of brain tumors and tumor recurrence. J Nucl Med 2011;52(10):1585–600.
10. Buchbender C, Heusner TA, Lauenstein TC, et al. Oncologic PET/MRI, Part 1: tumors of the brain, head and neck, chest, abdomen, and pelvis. J Nucl Med 2012;53(6):928–38.
11. Shao Y, Cherry SR, Farahani K, et al. Simultaneous PET and MR imaging. Phys Med Biol 1997;42(10):1965–70.
12. Judenhofer MS, Wehrl HF, Newport DF, et al. Simultaneous PET-MRI: a new approach for functional and-morphological imaging. Nat Med 2008;14(4):459–65.
13. Wehrl HF, Sauter AW, Judenhofer MS, et al. Combined PET/MR imaging—technology and applications. Technol Cancer Res Treat 2011;9(1):5–20.
14. Delso G, Furst S, Jakoby B, et al. Performance measurements of the Siemens mMR integrated whole-body PET/MR scanner. J Nucl Med 2011; 52(12):1914–22.
15. Pichler BJ, Kolb A, Nagele T, et al. PET/MRI: paving the way for the next generation of clinical multimodality imaging applications. J Nucl Med 2010; 51(3):333–6.
16. Judenhofer MS, Catana C, Swann BK, et al. PET/MR images acquired with a compact MR-compatible PET detector in a 7-T magnet. Radiology 2007; 244(3):807–14.
17. Schlemmer HP, Pichler BJ, Schmand M, et al. Simultaneous MR/PET imaging of the human brain: feasibility study. Radiology 2008;248(3):1028–35.
18. Herzog H, Pietrzyk U, Shah NJ, et al. The current state, challenges and perspectives of MR-PET. Neuroimage 2010;49(3):2072–82.
19. Zaidi H, Ojha N, Morich M, et al. Design and performance evaluation of a whole-body ingenuity TF PET-MRI system. Phys Med Biol 2011;56(10):3091–106.
20. Holdsworth SJ, Bammer R. Magnetic resonance imaging techniques: fMRI, DWI, and PWI. Semin Neurol 2008;28(4):395–406.
21. Cho ZH, Son YD, Kim HK, et al. A fusion PET-MRI system with a high-resolution research tomograph-PET and ultra-high field 7.0 T-MRI for the molecular-genetic imaging of the brain. Proteomics 2008;8(6): 1302–23.
22. Zaidi H, Schoenahl F, Ratib O. Geneva PET/CT facility: design considerations and performance characteristics of two commercial (Biograph 16/64) scanners. Eur J Nucl Med Mol Imaging 2007; 34(Suppl 2):S166.
23. Zaidi H, Montandon M-L, Assal F. Structure-function based quantitative brain image analysis. PET Clin 2010;5(2):155–68.
24. Zaidi H, Del Guerra A. An outlook on future design of hybrid PET/MRI systems. Med Phys 2011;38(10): 5667–89.
25. Mollet P, Keereman V, Clementel E, et al. Simultaneous MR-compatible emission and transmission imaging for PET using time-of-flight information. IEEE Trans Med Imaging 2012;31(9):1734–42.
26. Zaidi H. Is MR-guided attenuation correction a viable option for dual-modality PET/MR imaging? Radiology 2007;244(3):639–42.
27. Hofmann M, Pichler B, Schölkopf B, et al. Towards quantitative PET/MRI: a review of MR-based attenuation correction techniques. Eur J Nucl Med Mol Imaging 2009;36(Suppl 1):93–104.
28. Zaidi H, Montandon ML, Slosman DO. Magnetic resonance imaging-guided attenuation and scatter corrections in three-dimensional brain positron emission tomography. Med Phys 2003;30(5):937–48.
29. Zaidi H, Montandon ML, Meikle S. Strategies for attenuation compensation in neurological PET studies. Neuroimage 2007;34(2):518–41.
30. Catana C, van der Kouwe A, Benner T, et al. Toward implementing an MRI-based PET attenuation-correction method for neurologic studies on the

MR-PET brain prototype. J Nucl Med 2010;51(9): 1431–8.

31. Keereman V, Fierens Y, Broux T, et al. MRI-based attenuation correction for PET/MRI using ultrashort echo time sequences. J Nucl Med 2010;51(5):812–8.

32. Montandon ML, Zaidi H. Atlas-guided non-uniform attenuation correction in cerebral 3D PET imaging. Neuroimage 2005;25(1):278–86.

33. Hofmann M, Bezrukov I, Mantlik F, et al. MRI-based attenuation correction for whole-body PET/MRI: quantitative evaluation of segmentation- and atlas-based methods. J Nucl Med 2011;52(9):1392–9.

34. Marshall HR, Prato FS, Deans L, et al. Variable lung density consideration in attenuation correction of whole-body PET/MRI. J Nucl Med 2012;53(6): 977–84.

35. Chang T, Clark J, Mawlawi O. A novel approach for the attenuation correction of PET data in PET/MR systems. Med Phys 2012;39(6):3644.

36. Dogdas B, Shattuck DW, Leahy RM. Segmentation of skull and scalp in 3-D human MRI using mathematical morphology. Hum Brain Mapp 2005;26(4): 273–85.

37. Qi J, Leahy RM. Iterative reconstruction techniques in emission computed tomography. Phys Med Biol 2006;51(15):R541–78.

38. Reader AJ, Zaidi H. Advances in PET image reconstruction. PET Clin 2007;2(2):173–90.

39. Tang J, Rahmim A. Bayesian PET image reconstruction incorporating anato-functional joint entropy. Phys Med Biol 2009;54(23):7063–75.

40. Zaidi H, Ruest T, Schoenahl F, et al. Comparative assessment of statistical brain MR image segmentation algorithms and their impact on partial volume correction in PET. Neuroimage 2006;32(4): 1591–607.

41. Matsuda H, Ohnishi T, Asada T, et al. Correction for partial-volume effects on brain perfusion SPECT in healthy men. J Nucl Med 2003;44(8):1243–52.

42. Wang H, Fei B. An MR image-guided, voxel-based partial volume correction method for PET images. Med Phys 2012;39(1):179–95.

43. Shidahara M, Tsoumpas C, Hammers A, et al. Functional and structural synergy for resolution recovery and partial volume correction in brain PET. Neuroimage 2009;44(2):340–8.

44. Le Pogam A, Hatt M, Descourt P, et al. Evaluation of a 3D local multiresolution algorithm for the correction of partial volume effects in positron emission tomography. Med Phys 2011;38(9):4920–3.

45. Daou D. Respiratory motion handling is mandatory to accomplish the high-resolution PET destiny. Eur J Nucl Med Mol Imaging 2008;35(11):1961–70.

46. van der Kouwe AJ, Benner T, Dale AM. Real-time rigid body motion correction and shimming using cloverleaf navigators. Magn Reson Med 2006; 56(5):1019–32.

47. Chun SY, Reese TG, Ouyang J, et al. MRI-based nonrigid motion correction in simultaneous PET/MRI. J Nucl Med 2012;53(8):1284–91.

48. Tsoumpas C, Mackewn JE, Halsted P, et al. Simultaneous PET-MR acquisition and MR-derived motion fields for correction of non-rigid motion in PET. Ann Nucl Med 2010;24(10):745–50.

49. Catana C, Benner T, van der Kouwe A, et al. MRI-assisted PET motion correction for neurologic studies in an integrated MR-PET scanner. J Nucl Med 2011;52(1):154–61.

50. Waldman AD, Jackson A, Price SJ, et al. Quantitative imaging biomarkers in neuro-oncology. Nat Rev Clin Oncol 2009;6(8):445–54.

51. Garibotto V, Heinzer S, Vulliemoz S, et al. Clinical applications of hybrid PET/MR in neuroimaging. Clin Nucl Med 2012 in press.

52. Heinzel A, Stock S, Langen KJ, et al. Cost-effectiveness analysis of amino acid PET-guided surgery for supratentorial high-grade gliomas. J Nucl Med 2012;53(4):552–8.

53. Zaidi H, El Naqa I. PET-guided delineation of radiation therapy treatment volumes: a survey of image segmentation techniques. Eur J Nucl Med Mol Imaging 2010;37(11):2165–87.

54. Weber DC, Zilli T, Buchegger F, et al. [(18)F]Fluoroethyltyrosine- positron emission tomography-guided radiotherapy for high-grade glioma. Radiat Oncol 2008;3(1):44.

55. Vees H, Senthamizhchelvan S, Miralbell R, et al. Assessment of various strategies for 18F-FET PET-guided delineation of target volumes in high-grade glioma patients. Eur J Nucl Med Mol Imaging 2009;36(2):182–93.

56. Weber WA, Wester HJ, Grosu AL, et al. O-(2-[F-18] fluoroethyl)-L-tyrosine and L-[methyl-C-11]methionine uptake in brain tumours: initial results of a comparative study. Eur J Nucl Med 2000;27(5): 542–9.

57. Grosu AL, Weber WA, Riedel E, et al. L-(methyl-11C) methionine positron emission tomography for target delineation in resected high-grade gliomas before radiotherapy. Int J Radiat Oncol Biol Phys 2005; 63(1):64–74.

58. Grosu AL, Weber WA, Franz M, et al. Reirradiation of recurrent high-grade gliomas using amino acid PET (SPECT)/CT/MRI image fusion to determine gross tumor volume for stereotactic fractionated radiotherapy. Int J Radiat Oncol Biol Phys 2005;63(2): 511–9.

59. Galldiks N, Langen KJ, Holy R, et al. Assessment of treatment response in patients with glioblastoma using O-(2-18F-Fluoroethyl)-L-Tyrosine PET in comparison to MRI. J Nucl Med 2012;53(7):1048–57.

60. Piroth MD, Holy R, Pinkawa M, et al. Prognostic impact of postoperative, pre-irradiation F-18-fluoroethyl-L-tyrosine uptake in glioblastoma patients

treated with radiochemotherapy. Radiother Oncol 2011;99(2):218–24.

61. Krohn KA, Link JM, Mason RP. Molecular imaging of hypoxia. J Nucl Med 2008;49(Suppl 2):129S–48S.

62. Carlin S, Humm JL. PET of hypoxia: current and future perspectives. J Nucl Med 2012;53(8):1171–4.

63. Vaupel P, Hockel M, Mayer A. Detection and characterization of tumor hypoxia using pO2 histography. Antioxid Redox Signal 2007;9(8):1221–35.

64. Chitneni SK, Palmer GM, Zalutsky MR, et al. Molecular imaging of hypoxia. J Nucl Med 2011;52(2):165–8.

65. Ling CC, Humm J, Larson S, et al. Towards multidimensional radiotherapy (MD-CRT): biological imaging and biological conformality. Int J Radiat Oncol Biol Phys 2000;47(3):551–60.

66. Spence AM, Muzi M, Swanson KR, et al. Regional hypoxia in glioblastoma multiforme quantified with [18F]fluoromisonidazole positron emission tomography before radiotherapy: correlation with time to progression and survival. Clin Cancer Res 2008;14(9):2623–30.

67. Bloom HJ. Intracranial tumors: response and resistance to therapeutic endeavors, 1970–1980. Int J Radiat Oncol Biol Phys 1982;8(7):1083–113.

# Index

*Note:* Page numbers of article titles are in **boldface** type.

## A

[$^{11}$C]-Acetate, 129, 139–140
American College of Radiology recommendations, for glioma imaging, 124
Amino acid tracers, 136–137, 202–203, 227–228. *See also specific tracers.*
Amino acid transporters, 136–137
Antiangiogenic therapy, for gliomas, MR imaging in, **163–182**
Apparent diffusion coefficient, 173–179, 184
Attenuation correction, in PET/MR imaging, 221–224

## B

Bevacizumab, imaging appearance with, 133, 163–182
Biograph PET/MR imaging system, 221
Biopsy
    FET PET For, 156
    for gliomas, 120–121
Blood-brain barrier, tumor and tracer penetration of, 131–133, 139
Bombesin analogues, 141
Brain tumors. *See also specific types, eg,* Gliomas.
    classification of, 130–131
    extra-axial, 130–131
    intra-axial, 130–131
    metastatic. *See* Metastatic brain tumors.
    MR imaging for. *See* MR imaging; PET/MR imaging.
    parametric response mapping in, **201–217**
    PET/MR imaging for. *See* PET/MR imaging.
    tracers for. *See* Tracers.
    treatment response evaluation for, **147–162, 201–217**
BrainPET dedicated instrument, 220–221

## C

Carcinoid tumors, tracers for, 140–141
CHO ([$^{11}$C]-Choline), 129, 132, 138–139
Choline transporters, 138–139
CIMPLE maps, 178–179
Computed tomography, PET with, versus PET/MR imaging, 220
Contrast agents
    for gliomas, for biopsy, 120–121
    for MR imaging, 173, 189–190

Copper(II) diacetyl-2,3-bis(N4-methyl-3-thiosemicarbazone)([60/62/64Cu]-ASTM), 129, 132, 137–138, 228–229

## D

1-(2'-Deoxy-2'[$^{18}$F]fluoro-β-D-arabinofuranosyl)thymine (FMAU), 135
Diffusion MR imaging, 173–179
Diffusion-tensor imaging, 185–188
Diffusion-weighted MR imaging, 184–185
DOTATATE, $^{177}$Lu-labeled, 141
DOTATATE,$^{68}$Gallium-labeled, 129, 140–141
DOTATOC, $^{68}$Gallium-labeled, 129, 140–141
Dynamic contrast-enhanced MR imaging, 173, 189–190
Dynamic susceptibilities contrast MR imaging, 169–173, 189–190

## F

FCHO ([$^{18}$F]fluorocholine (N,N-dimethyl)ethanol ammonium), 138–139
FDG ([$^{18}$F]-fluorodeoxyglucose), 129, 133–134, 202
    action of, 133
    for gliomas, 118–120, 122–123
    for parametric response mapping, 203, 206–209
    for PET/MR imaging, 220
    versus acetate tracers, 140
    versus choline tracers, 138
    whole-body, 131
FDOPA ([$^{18}$F]fluoro-3,4-dihydroxy-L-phenylalanine), 129, 135–136, 202–203
    for parametric response mapping, 206, 210–211
FET ([$^{18}$F]-fluoroethyltyrosine), 129, 136, 141, **147–162,** 202–203
    chemical structure of, 148
    pharmacokinetics of, 148–149
    uptake of, 148–149
FET ([$^{18}$F]-fluoroethyltyrosine) PET
    for biopsy, 156
    for gliomas, 119–123
    for malignant transformation, 154–156
    for progression, 156–158
    for pseudoprogression, 156–158
    for treatment response evaluation, 158–159
    image analysis for, 149–150
    imaging protocols for, 149, 151
    indications for, 148

PET Clin 8 (2013) 233–235
http://dx.doi.org/10.1016/S1556-8598(13)00011-4
1556-8598/13/$ – see front matter © 2013 Elsevier Inc. All rights reserved.

Printed and bound by CPI Group (UK) Ltd, Croydon, CR0 4YY

03/10/2024

01040347-0006